hea   for
p   cy

amanda grant

healthy eating for
pregnancy

**the complete guide to a healthy diet
before, during and after pregnancy**

MITCHELL BEAZLEY

Healthy Eating for Pregnancy
by Amanda Grant

First published in Great Britain in 2001 by Mitchell Beazley, an imprint of Octopus Publishing Group Limited,
2–4 Heron Quays, London E14 4JP.
Reprinted 2002, 2003
© Octopus Publishing Group Limited 2001
Text © Amanda Grant 2001

A CIP catalogue record for this book is available from the British Library.

ISBN 1 84000 739 7

Commissioning Editor: Rebecca Spry
Executive Art Editor: Phil Ormerod
Managing Editor: Emma Rice
Design: Miranda Harvey
Editors: Jo Richardson, Jamie Ambrose
Counsultant Nutritionist: Tanya Carr
Production: Jessame Emms
Index: John Noble
Photography: William Reavell

Typeset in Helvetica Neue
Printed and bound by Toppan Printing Company in China

contents

6 pre-conception diet
8   pre-conception care
12   fertility: what to eat
26   fertility: what to avoid

32 pregnancy diet
34   pregnancy care
40   pregnancy nutrition

62 pregnancy and food safety
64   foods & safety
76   foods & comfort
85   drugs & safety

88 pregnancy recipes
90   three meals a day
91   breakfasts
100   lunches
112   suppers
124   desserts
126   snacks

132 breastfeeding diet
134   breastfeeding care
137   breastfeeding nutrition
140   breastfeeding myths

141   further reading
144   index

these symbols are used in the recipe section:

suitable for freezing

suitable for toddlers

prepare in advance

preconception diet

preconception care

At conception, if both parents have taken similar care and attention with their health, they are more likely to produce a healthy baby.

preparing for pregnancy

In order to create a healthy baby, why not consider applying the principles used in organic farming?

Organic farmers prepare the soil with natural nutrients over many years and avoid processed chemicals. This results in strong, vigorous, healthy plants which are able to resist diseases and pests. All the vitamins, minerals, enzymes and essential nutrients are in balance.

At conception, if both parents have taken similar care and attention with their health, they are more likely to produce a healthy baby.

Preconception care is the term given to the method of bringing both parents as close to optimum health as possible *before* they try to conceive. It creates the healthiest physical environment for a growing embryo.

Preconception care has the benefit of maximizing the chances of a healthy sperm, ova, and uterus; in turn, this helps to foster a healthy pregnancy.

history of preconception care

Preconception care has been around for many centuries – there are even references to it in the Bible: "And the angel of the Lord appeared unto the woman, and said unto her: '...thou shalt conceive, and bear a son. Now therefore beware, I pray thee, and drink not wine nor strong drink, and eat not any unclean thing.'" (Ref. 1.1)

In 1978, the Foresight Association for the Promotion of Preconceptual Care was established in the UK to help couples prepare for pregnancy – to give them the best possible chance of producing healthy babies. The association has two main objectives. The first is to safeguard the health of any unborn child by promoting preconception care, while the second is to promote the study of aspects of the environment upon preconception health. For more information about the association, or to speak to one of their clinicians, see "Useful Addresses", page 143.

Thousands of much-wanted babies are stillborn or miscarried each year, and many are born frail, often as a result of a lack of information about preconception care. Foresight's objective is to pass on this knowledge to help all parents achieve a healthy, full-term pregnancy. Some experts believe that it is possible to reduce, and in many cases, eliminate, infertility, pregnancy, and birth problems.

conception problems

It is often too late to prevent many problems once a woman knows that she is pregnant.

Alcohol and smoking are at their most hazardous during the earliest stages of pregnancy, when cell division is at its highest. It is therefore important that if a woman decides to become pregnant, she should avoid these substances from the first opportunity. Having said that, if you discover you are already pregnant, it is obviously still advisable to stop smoking and drinking as soon as possible.

Approximately one in six couples will have some difficulty conceiving. About one in 10 couples will take more than a year to conceive and one in 20 more than two years. Even in the most fertile couples, the chance of becoming pregnant in each menstrual cycle is only 25 percent (Ref. 1.2).

In order to prepare fully for conception, the issues in the following pages need to be considered.

preconception nutrition

...it is advised by experts that couples start putting good nutrition into practice at least four months – the longer, the better – before trying to conceive.

"We are what we eat", as the saying goes. We need top-quality "fuel" in order for our bodies to function properly and to produce healthy eggs or sperm. In other words, good nutrition is essential for good health.

The food we eat has an impact on every cell in our bodies. Eating healthily can help women to conceive and give birth to a healthy baby – *see* pages 34–61 for more information about healthy eating.

Good nutrition for men helps ensure healthy sperm and sexual activity. Poor nutrition in women can lead to fertility problems as highlighted by birth-rate studies during famines (*Ref. 1.3*).

In fact, the inability to reproduce can be one of the first signs of imperfect nutrition. This vital link between nutrition and foetal development has been researched by a number of scientists. The work of Isobel Jennings, Weston Price, E J Underwood, Donald Oberleas, Donald Caldwell, Lucille Hurley, Bert Vallee, and many others has drawn attention to the role played by a lack of nutrients in reproductive problems under experimental conditions.

Such studies have found that, in many cases, almost all the commonly seen birth defects can be reduced or eliminated by changing the diet .

It is advised by experts that couples start putting good nutrition into practice at least four months – the longer, the better – before trying to conceive. This will at least give the body a chance to correct any nutritional deficiencies. This four-month "minimum" period is also recommended because it takes at least three months for men to produce a new batch of sperm and women's eggs to mature, ready for ovulation.

You might like to ask your GP to refer you to a state-registered dietician or registered nutritionist, specializing in diet for preconception and pregnancy. He or she will be able to assess your nutrient intake as well as point out any signs of nutrient deficiencies, and advise appropriate action.

At the end of the four months, the assessment should be repeated. You will then be given a maintenance programme to adhere to until you conceive and ideally for life! (*Ref. 1.4*).

A well-balanced vegetarian diet is
extremely healthy for all life stages, including
preconception and pregnancy...

organic

There is a growing awareness of
the benefits of eating organic food.
For Instance, research carried out
in 1994 by the Department of
Occupational Medicine in
Denmark found that men who
regularly ate organic food had
twice the sperm count of those on
a conventional diet. It is probably
just a matter of time before the
health benefits of organic foods
are proven scientifically.

vegetarian & vegan

A well-balanced vegetarian diet can
provide the nutritional and calorific
requirements for fertility. A poorly
planned vegetarian diet, just like a
poorly planned diet that includes
meat, can result in decreased
fertility (*Ref. 1.5*).

Vegans may take longer to
conceive, according to *Nutrition and
Pregnancy: A Complete Guide from
Preconception to Post-delivery* by
Judith E Brown (*Ref. 1.6*). The
author found that, while vegans do
not tend to be infertile, they may
take longer to conceive because a
high-plant diet appears to increase
menstrual cycle length, causing less
frequent ovulation. This is no cause
for concern, however; it is simply
something for vegans to keep in
mind when trying to conceive.

fertility:
what to eat

fats

Contrary to popular belief, not all fats are bad. However, before reaching for the chocolate and cream cakes lurking menacingly in the back of the fridge, it is worth bearing in mind that most of us in the UK eat too much of the wrong types of fat and not enough of the beneficial kind. Some of the "good" types of fats are known as "essential" fats, while those generally considered "bad" are known as "saturated fats". Chocolate and cream are in the "bad" category!

There are two fatty acids that the body cannot make; they must be sourced from what we eat.

essential fats

Fat is made up of substances called fatty acids. There are two fatty acids that the body cannot make; they must be sourced from what we eat. Known as essential (polyunsaturated) fatty acids (EFAs) (*see* page 44 for more details) these are called alpha-linolenic acid and linoleic acid. They are vital for good health.

We need EFAs to keep the body warm, the skin and arteries supple, and the hormones in balance. In fact, they have a significant effect on every system in the body, including reproduction.

From EFAs we produce beneficial substances called prostaglandins, which behave as hormones. If these become imbalanced, it may be difficult to conceive. However, this situation may be rectified in some people by increasing good sources of essential fats in the diet.

Also, sperm is rich in prostaglandins, which is why men will benefit from essential fats in the diet. Semen taken from poor sperm samples has been found to lack adequate amount of these beneficial prostaglandins (*Ref 1.7*).

Essential fats are found in oils, oily fish, nuts and seeds. It is possible to maintain an acceptable daily intake of essential fatty acids by eating a handful of seeds and nuts, or by using good-quality oils in cooking and dressings. It is also advisable to include oily fish such as mackerel and sardines in our diet.

saturated fats

Even though they stimulate oestrogen, saturated fats can adversely affect fertility. A diet high in saturated fats can also restrict the usage of the EFAs in the body.

Saturated fats tend to be mainly solid at room temperature. They are mainly sourced from animals, so you may need to restrict your intake of foods like dairy produce (including butter, eggs, full-fat milk, yogurt and cheese) and meats.

fibre

It has been found that a healthy, high-fibre diet will reduce high levels of toxic metals, such as lead.

An adequate supply of fibre in the diet helps the human body to achieve three main objectives.

It ensures that nutrients are absorbed in a systematic, steady fashion, and helps to produce substances that fight against "free-radical" damage (free radicals are naturally occurring oxygen molecules that damage human and animal tissue and are thought to play a key role in the aging process).

In addition, fibre keeps the bowels healthy and prevents constipation. This is particularly important for fertility because women need to get rid of chemicals, pesticides, heavy toxic metals, and other toxins that may have an adverse affect on their reproductive systems. It has been found that a healthy, high-fibre diet can help reduce high levels of toxic metals, such as lead.(Ref. 1.9).

Women also need to excrete old oestrogens (female hormones) from their bodies in order to help keep their reproductive systems in optimum balance. Fibre contained in whole grains and fruit and vegetables enables the body to do this.

To increase fibre intake, eat plenty of fresh fruit, vegetables (cooked and, whenever possible, raw), wholegrains (brown rice, wholemeal bread, oats, wholegrain crackers, wholemeal pasta, etc.), beans, nuts, and seeds.

carbohydrates

It is advisable to eat as many complex carbohydrates as possible and as few simple carbohydrates as possible.

Like fats, carbohydrates provide the body with energy. There are two types of carbohydrates: simple and complex. Simple carbohydrates (sugars) are found in foods such as cakes, biscuits and jams, as well as honey. Complex carbohydrates are found in wholegrain foods and wholemeal flours. Good examples include wholewheat pasta, brown rice and potatoes.

It is advisable to eat as many complex carbohydrates as possible and as few simple carbohydrates as possible. There are a few reasons for this: simple carbohydrates are often found in foods high in sugars and fats but containing very little else. Consequently, these foods are not very nutrient dense. If your diet relies heavily on these foods, you may run the risk of not having a sufficient supply of all the essential nutrients.

Also, if eaten on their own, simple carbohydrates can cause blood-sugar levels to fluctuate, which is not advisable as this may affect hormonal cycles. If you do eat simple carbohydrates, it is advisable to combine them with the complex variety to reduce any blood-sugar swings. Better still, aim to avoid sugar or sugar-based snacks altogether.

protein

A low intake of protein can reduce chances of conception, so women must make sure that they eat a good range of high-quality protein foods. As most of us gain much of our required protein from meat and dairy products, vegetarians – and vegans even more so – need to pay particular attention to this aspect of their diet. For more information about protein and good vegetarian sources of protein, *see* page 47.

zinc

Zinc is important to the body for a number of reasons. It helps growth, aids healing, assists in coping with stress, promotes a healthy brain and nervous system – particularly in a growing foetus – helps ensure that energy supplies are both stable and sustained, and boosts our ability to maintain a healthy immune system.

Much research has been carried out on zinc and its effects on the human body. There is a fair weight of evidence to suggest that it is important for fertility in both men and women.

...research has been carried out on zinc and its effects on the human body. There is a fair weight of evidence to suggest that it is important for fertility in both men and women.

...if levels of
zinc are not at
an optimum,
conception is
difficult; there are
also risks that
any babies which
are conceived
may have a low
birth weight and
other possible
complications.

males

The main conclusions of the
numerous studies carried out on
zinc and male fertility are that zinc is
needed for the proper development
of sperm (Ref 1.8). In addition, if
there is a lack of zinc, the sperm
may not be able to penetrate the
egg (Ref 1.9). Zinc is also necessary
for the production of the
reproductive hormones oestrogen
and progesterone (Ref 1.10). Finally,
zinc plays a vital role in cell division.

females

As far as the effects of zinc on
the female reproductive system
is concerned, the Foresight
Association has found that many
women having difficulty conceiving
show high levels of copper and low
levels of zinc. It has also been found
that the contraceptive pill can inhibit
the absorption of zinc. In addition, if
levels of zinc are not at an optimum,
conception is difficult; there are also
risks that any babies which are
conceived may have a low birth
weight and other possible
complications (Ref 1.11).

As a result of these issues,
it is important to ensure that
adequate levels of zinc are present
in the diet both before and at the
time of conception.

Zinc levels can be improved by
eating zinc-rich foods. Such sources
include lamb, turkey, sardines, hard
cheeses, wheatgerm and wholegrain
cereals, pulses such as lentils,
beans and chickpeas, green
vegetables such as watercress,
spinach and peas, and fruits such
as dried apricots and figs.

manganese

Like zinc, manganese is needed to help prevent infertility in both men and women. It is also used to help control blood-sugar levels, assist with cell protection and the formation of bones, skin, and cartilage.

Low manganese levels have also been linked to decreased libido in both sexes. In addition, babies born to mothers with low manganese levels may be more prone to birth defects.

A well-balanced diet is likely to provide sufficient manganese. Good specific sources of it include tropical fruits, nuts, seeds and wholegrains.

selenium

Good levels of selenium are also essential for the healthy development of sperm. Blood-selenium levels have been found to be lower in men with low sperm counts.

Selenium is an antioxidant – a group of substances believed to reduce the risk of cancer, heart disease, and other age-related diseases.

Selenium can also help to prevent birth defects and miscarriages. It can help protect against poisoning from heavy toxic metals (*see pages 26-7 and 30*).

Good levels of selenium are also essential for the healthy development of sperm. Blood-selenium levels have been found to be lower in men with low sperm counts (*Ref 1.12*).

Selenium is found in nuts such as Brazil nuts; seeds such as sunflower seeds; milk; wholemeal bread (but only if made with flour grown in selenium-rich soil), cheese, eggs, chicken, shellfish, and fish.

folic acid

There are a number of reasons why women need folic acid in their diets. First of all, it helps to create healthy blood cells; insufficient supplies can result in anaemia. Secondly, it helps the body absorb iron.

Folic acid is also needed in the production of genetic material. It is important in fertility as well as during pregnancy, and it can help to prevent spina bifida (see page 56).

The human body cannot store large quantities of folic acid; in fact, we can only store a supply that is sufficient for a maximum of two or three months. It is therefore important to eat foods rich in folic acid as part of the daily diet.

Good sources of folic acid include green, leafy vegetables; asparagus; oranges; and wheatgerm. However, the content of folic acid in food tends to reduce over time; the longer they are left after picking, the lower the folic acid content. We need to eat foods as fresh as possible and keep cooking times as short as possible in order to gain the maximum benefit from the nutritive value of these foods. Salads, stir-fries, and steamed vegetables are all great ways of enjoying folic-acid-rich vegetables.

The contraceptive pill and other forms of medication (aspirin and indigestion remedies) as well as alcohol may decrease the amount of folic acid stored in the body.

In addition to eating folic-acid-rich foods, the British Department of Health recommends that women planning a pregnancy should take supplements of 400 micrograms (mcg) of folic acid a day for three months prior to conception and throughout the first three months of pregnancy.

The human body cannot store large quantities of folic acid; in fact, we can only store a supply that is sufficient for a maximum of two or three months.

B$_{12}$

Vitamin B$_{12}$ has many roles to play in general well-being. It is required to develop and maintain a healthy nervous system. We need it to help with the digestion of food and the conversion of food into energy. It is also necessary to produce red blood cells.

Lack of this vitamin may result in a form of anaemia which is associated with infertility. Low levels of B$_{12}$ can also contribute towards a low sperm count. Studies have demonstrated the potential of vitamin B$_{12}$ for increasing male fertility (*Ref 1.13*).

Women in particular need to make sure that their diets are rich in vitamin B$_{12}$. Good sources are primarily of animal origin, including milk and cheese. Other foods include oily fish such as sardines and pilchards. Vegans need to pay particular attention to their intake of B$_{12}$.

B$_6$ (pyridoxine)

We need vitamin B$_6$ to help convert protein into energy and aid with the functioning of both the nervous and immune systems.

Women who have trouble conceiving have been known to benefit from increasing their intake of vitamin B$_6$. In some women, B$_6$ has been shown to increase levels of progesterone, a female hormone needed to maintain a healthy womb lining and to support growth of a fertilized egg (*Ref. 1.14*).

The best way to increase your vitamin B6 levels is to eat vitamin B6-rich foods. These include dark green leafy vegetables, nuts, lentils, peanuts, bananas, and melons.

Women who have trouble conceiving have been known to benefit from increasing their intake of vitamin B$_6$.

vitamin c

Vitamin C, a powerful antioxidant, is needed for growth and health of body tissue, and it is necessary for the healing of wounds. It can also protect the sperm and its DNA from damage (*Ref 1.15*). Studies have shown how male fertility has been improved when men increase their vitamin C intake (*Ref 1.16*). When sperm enter a woman's body, antibodies directed against them cause the sperm to clump together, which renders them less likely to fertilize the egg. Vitamin C helps to reduce this process of agglutination.

Vitamin C is a water-soluble vitamin that cannot be stored in the body in large amounts. If we consume too much, our bodies will just get rid of it. We rely on our diet for vitamin C, unlike nearly all other animals who are able to make the vitamin themselves. Fruits and vegetables are the main sources of this vitamin. If we eat the recommended five servings of fresh fruits and vegetables a day, we should be eating enough to get our daily requirement. Particularly good fruits include strawberries, oranges, kiwi fruit, blackcurrants, mangoes, papayas, lychees and peaches. Good vegetable sources include red peppers, spinach, watercress, and peas.

vitamin A

As well as being necessary for growth, healthy skin, hair and vision, vitamin A is essential for reproduction. It maintains healthy tissues that line all external and internal surfaces of the body, including the linings of the vagina and uterus. During pregnancy, it is also needed by the developing baby.

It is therefore important that, both before and after conception, women receive a good intake of vitamin A. If you eat a well-balanced diet, you should receive enough vitamin A from your food. Good animal sources include milk, cheese, and egg yolks.

Betacarotene, a substance found in orange, yellow, and green vegetables, is converted into vitamin A in the body.

Vitamin A maintains healthy tissues that line all the external and internal surfaces of the body.

iron

We need iron for healthy blood and muscles. Iron is also known to have helped women with infertility problems.

We need iron for healthy blood and muscles. Iron is also known to have helped women with infertility problems (*Ref 1.17*). It is therefore advisable to include iron-rich foods in your daily diet.

Good sources of iron include lean meat, eggs (during pregnancy, make sure that these are properly cooked), and green leafy vegetables such as spinach and broccoli. Iron in non-meat foods is not as easily absorbed by the body, so we need to eat more of these foods to gain the equivalent amount of iron.

Vitamin C aids in the absorption of iron, so it is also advisable to eat a good supply of foods rich in this vitamin at the same time.

Drinks such as tea and coffee contain tannins which can inhibit the absorption of iron, so it is advisable to keep these drinks to an absolute minimum. This is sensible advise for good general health as well. See page 28 for information about caffeine and fertility.

vitamin E

Vitamin E has been shown to be of benefit to both male and female fertility.

Like vitamins C and A, vitamin E is a powerful antioxidant. These substances have the ability to fight free radicals linked to cancer, coronary heart disease and infertility, which destroy cells and can speed up the ageing process.

Vitamin E has been shown to be of benefit to both male and female fertility and is of particular importance for those over 35. It is also necessary for the production of healthy sperm, and, along with zinc, manganese, and vitamin B12, is vital for a good sperm count. Vitamin E is also needed for the development and maintenance of strong cells, particularly in the blood.

It is therefore a good idea to make sure that your diet contains a good supply of vitamin E and other antioxidant vitamins. It is quite possible to receive adequate amounts of vitamin E from a well-balanced diet that includes such foods as mangoes, sweet potatoes, watercress, avocados, spinach, and vegetable oils such as olive oil.

organic foods

Some experts believe that eating an organic wholefood diet will help improve fertility. Some research is based on the work carried out by the Foresight Association (*see* "Useful addresses" page 143). Foresight has helped thousands of people to conceive healthy babies, including those who have failed IVF.

Part of the Foresight programme is based on eating a healthy, well-balanced diet composed of as much organic foods as possible. Just like many other experts, the Foresight organization states that it is better to eat organic foods that are free from pesticide residues than their non-organic equivalents, especially when trying to conceive.

There is also a school of thought that believes organic food may be better nutritionally, but this is still being researched.

Foresight stresses the dangers of environmental toxins, identifying at least 200 man-made chemicals for which there is evidence of

reproductive hazards. The association also stresses that eating organic foods will at least help to reduce the risks of some of these chemicals.

Surrey University undertook some research on Foresight's work and studied a group of 367 couples who enrolled on the Foresight programme due to number of different problems. Of these 367, 217 had infertility issues. Within one to three years, 327 of the group had successfully conceived healthy children. The success rate among the infertile couples in the group was 86 percent.

Eating organic food is just one of the recommendations made by Foresight; a considerable number of other factors also play a part in successful conception. *See* pages 38-39 for more information about organic foods.

There is also a school of thought that believes organic food may be better nutritionally, but this is still being researched.

staying healthy

Being underweight or overweight can have an affect on conception...

weight

Achieving and maintaining an ideal body weight is important both to general health and fertility. Being underweight or overweight can have an affect on conception – see pages 78-9, or consult a registered nutritionist, dietician, or your doctor for more information on ideal weights.

In addition, research has indicated that excessive dieting and overeating can contribute to infertility problems.

If women are overweight, they can stop ovulating. Studies have shown that losing even a little weight can be sufficient to increase fertility by stimulating ovulation, improving hormone balance and making periods more regular.

Consequently, experts advise achieving an ideal body weight by eating a healthy and nutritious diet (see pages 34-61). Women should also aim to maintain that weight for as long as possible prior to conception. This allows their bodies the chance to achieve the balance of hormones that will maximize the chances of conceiving (Ref 1.18).

contraceptive pill

The pill interferes with the hormone system to prevent pregnancy. Bear in mind that it may take your body a little time to start producing these hormones again once you have stopped taking the pill (Ref 1.19). Foresight usually recommends mineral testing and readjustment after the use of this form of contraception (Ref 1.20).

fertility:
what to avoid

There is much evidence to suggest that toxic metals can be harmful to the body and have a negative effect on fertility levels.

toxic metals

Toxic metals are defined as "those elements not recognized as having an essential function and known to have well-documented deleterious effects" (*Ref. 1.21*).

There is much evidence to suggest that toxic metals can be harmful to the body and may have a negative effect on fertility levels. The key toxic metals on which research has been focused include the following.

lead

Lead which comes, for example, from water that flows through lead pipes, was used in the past to induce an abortion (*Ref. 1.22*).

Men exposed to high levels of lead in the workplace have been found to be at risk of low sperm counts, with a greater number of sperm likely to be misshapen and less mobile (*Ref. 1.23*).

mercury

Mercury is found in pesticides, fungicides, fish, dental fillings, and industrial processes. Female dental assistants and female dentists exposed to mercury through the fillings they handle have been found to be less fertile than females who don't come into contact with the metal (*Ref. 1.24*).

The UK Department of Health recommends that pregnant women do not have mercury fillings put in place during pregnancy.

cadmium

Cadmium is an inorganic poison present in tobacco smoke, processed foods, manufacturing industries, shellfish from polluted waters, and galvanized containers. It accumulates in the body, and blocks nutrients such as zinc, which is critical for both male and female fertility.

Cadmium blocks nutrients such as zinc, which is critical for both male and female fertility.

aluminium

Aluminium, found in indigestion tablets, cookware or foil, canned drinks, dried milk substitutes, and deodorants, can be absorbed by the skin.

copper

Copper can be both toxic and beneficial, depending on the amount of exposure to it. Your body absorbs copper from water pipes, contraceptive coils, swimming pools, and jewellery. Copper can increase its concentration in the body after hormonal treatments, such as the contraceptive pill or fertility drugs.

assessing your toxins

In order to assess the levels of toxic metals present in the body, it is worth contacting Foresight (*see* "Useful Addresses", page 143). The association can carry out a hair analysis or arrange a personal consultation with a nutritional practitioner so that tests can be organized and a plan of action structured to your own individual needs. Alternatively, contact a registered nutritionist or dietician.

A nutritionist will help identify the source of contamination, which will then need to be avoided if possible. In addition, Foresight may recommend taking specific nutrients such as antioxidants (vitamin C, for example) to help eliminate toxins from the body.

The liver detoxifies the body by combining harmful substances (e.g., chemicals, drugs, alcohol, heavy toxic metals) with less harmful substances, which are then excreted by the kidneys. Making sure the liver is working as healthily and as efficiently as possible will help eliminate heavy toxins and other unwanted substances. Seek advice (as above) on the best ways of doing this.

caffeine

Caffeine is more widely used than many people expect. In addition to tea and coffee, caffeine is also present in chocolate, soft drinks and medicines – particularly some widely available headache remedies.

Caffeine is a diuretic, causing its user to pass more urine than normal and potentially flushing away vital nutrients that are important to fertility.

Ideally, aim to eliminate caffeine altogether or reduce your intake of it to the lowest possible level. This may be achieved gradually to reduce the unpleasant effects of withdrawal such as headaches, tiredness, or depression.

Caffeine is a diuretic, causing its user to pass more urine than normal and potentially flushing away vital nutrients that are important to fertility.

food additives

Food additives come in the form of preservatives and artificial colourings, flavourings and sweeteners, to name but a few. There are over 4,000 additives – both artificial and natural – in use in the UK. To date, very little research has been carried out on the effects of additives before and during pregnancy. Consequently, organizations such as the Foresight association recommend avoiding additives prior to conception. It is certainly a good idea to avoid all artificial additives if at all possible. Choosing organic foods can go some way to helping achieve this.

alcohol

Most of us have heard that drinking and smoking while pregnant can be harmful to the baby. What most of us may not realize is that smoking and alcohol can reduce fertility.

Research has shown that drinking alcohol causes a decrease in sperm counts, and an increase in abnormal sperm (*Ref. 1.25*).

In addition, alcohol can prevent the absorption of nutrients such as zinc, which is regarded as one of the most important minerals for male virility.

Foetal alcohol syndrome (FAS) was originally defined by a group of medical researchers in the USA. It has now been more clearly defined by international research, and the abnormalities of a baby suffering from FAS range from being underweight and under-length at birth to having slow growth and a failure to thrive after birth even with special postnatal care. Additional potential problems include possible mental retardation and/or behavioural problems such as hyperactivity and extreme nervousness.

For maximum safety and optimum development in the child, Foresight (*see* page 9) advises a complete embargo on alcohol for both parents in the four months leading up to the intended conception, and for the mother throughout pregnancy and breastfeeding.

The UK Department of Health advises that women trying to become pregnant should drink no more than one or two units – a unit is one glass of wine or half a pint of beer – of alcohol once or twice a week and should avoid heavy drinking sessions. The same advice comes from the UK's Health Development Agency.

In a study in Denmark, Dr Tina Kold Jensen and colleagues from the National University Hospital studied 430 Danish couples aged 20 to 35 years who were trying to have a baby for the first time. The results of the study were published in the *British Medical Journal*.

In this study, women who consumed an average of 11 to 15 drinks a week during a cycle had only a third of the chance of conceiving that month as women who avoided alcohol altogether. Moderate drinkers – those who had six to 10 drinks a week – were half as likely to conceive. Even light drinkers – those who had one to five drinks a week – cut their chances of becoming pregnant by a third.

If you are trying to conceive, it makes sense to refrain from drinking or at least limit your intake (*Ref 1.26*).

tobacco

When smoked, tobacco produces more than 4,000 compounds including carbon monoxide, oxides of nitrogen, ammonia, aromatic hydrocarbons, hydrogen cyanide, vinyl chloride, lead, and cadmium, in addition to nicotine.

Cigarette smoking has been linked to infertility problems in both women (*Refs 1.28 & 1.29*) and men (*Ref 1.27*).

Smoking has also been linked to problems in pregnancy and childbirth. Prematurity is seen to be higher in mothers who smoke compared to those who don't. Similarly, studies have found that smokers are more likely to give birth to children with all types of congenital malformations.

For example, the "Oxford Survey on Childhood Cancers", published in 1997 in the *British Journal of Cancer*, found that men who smoke when their partners don't still run a higher risk of fathering children who develop cancer. The survey stated that one in seven childhood cancers, including leukaemia and brain tumours, could be due to the father's smoking habits.

It is advisable to stop smoking at least four months prior to conception, and to avoid smoky atmospheres as much as possible.

It is advisable to stop smoking at least four months prior to conception.

drugs

The use of street drugs such as cocaine and marijuana has increased steadily over the years. Many drugs have been associated with infertility and, if taken during pregnancy, may bring about problems with the unborn baby's health and development. Babies born to mothers who have taken certain drugs during pregnancy can also suffer withdrawal symptoms (often severe).

Research indicates that if women take such drugs during pregnancy, they risk giving birth to babies with low birth weights or malformations, as well as being more prone to miscarriages and stillbirths (*Ref 1.30*).

If you are addicted to a street drug, seek professional help by talking to your doctor, who can then refer you to a specialist to help overcome the problem. It is recommended that women eliminate all drugs from their bodies at least four months before conception.

The Foresight Association (*see* page 9) also recommends avoiding the use of all over-the-counter drugs such as laxatives, painkillers, etc., where possible, before and during pregnancy. The association believes that by paying attention to your diet you can help to eliminate the need for this sort of medication.

It does not matter what the drug is; it will always have an unnatural effect on the body's biochemistry (*Ref 1.31*).

It does not matter what the drug is; it will always have an unnatural effect on the body's biochemistry.

excessive exercise

Everyone should aim to incorporate some form of exercise into his or her lifestyle to help keep bodies fit and healthy. Before and during pregnancy, this advice is no different. You should adapt your exercise routine to suit your base level of fitness

Excessive exercise – any exercise that places extreme physical stress on the body and lowers body fat to below what is needed to maintain normal menstrual function – is not advisable, either before and during pregnancy. Menstrual disorders have been reported in underweight athletic women and also in women with eating disorders such as anorexia nervosa.

Good forms of gentle exercise include swimming and yoga. For more information, contact the Active Birth Centre (*see* "Useful Addresses" page 143).

pregnancy diet

pregnancy care

eating during pregnancy

...many experts have been able to show a definite link between a newborn baby's health and its mother's diet during pregnancy.

During pregnancy, what you eat and drink will invariably affect the health and development of another little person.

Take the opportunity to have a thorough look at your diet and make any necessary changes to help reach your optimum health. If you are fit and healthy, there is a stronger chance that you will produce a fit and healthy baby. In the myriad studies on relationships between diet and pregnancy, many experts have been able to show a definite link between a newborn baby's health and its mother's diet during pregnancy.

During its time in the womb, a baby is completely dependent on its mother for the nutrients it needs to grow and develop. With most nutrients, the baby's needs tend to be met before the mother's. While this is good news for the developing baby, it is still important that expectant mothers achieve the recommended nutrient intakes from their diet to help prevent any problems with general health, such as brittle hair, bad teeth, sallow skin, etc.

Some mothers may experience challenges such as fatigue, morning sickness, cramps, anaemia, etc., many of which can be greatly reduced or even avoided altogether with a good diet.

To help you work towards a healthy diet, take a look at the following guidelines recommended by the Food Standards Agency. The rest of the chapter looks at a list of specific nutrients in detail.

- Enjoy your food. Don't give up any of the foods you enjoy most.
- Eat a variety of different foods. No one food contains all the nutrients needed in the right amounts, so eat a mixture of foods to get the right amount of a good range of nutrients.
- Choose foods from the following five food groups.
1   Bread, cereals and potatoes. This includes breakfast cereals, muesli, oats, pasta, noodles, sweet potatoes, and cornmeal.
2   Fruit and vegetables. This group includes salads, and fresh and frozen fruits.
3   Milk and dairy, e.g. yoghurt, milk, and cheese
4   Meat, fish, and alternatives, e.g. fresh and frozen fish, lamb, pork and beef, eggs, beans, lentils, and nuts.
5   Foods containing fat and sugar. Foods in this group include butter and oil, cakes, cookies, puddings, and other sweets.

Foods from the first four groups should be eaten every day, while foods in the fifth group are best not eaten too often or in large amounts. It is also important to choose a variety of foods from each group, rather than just eating the same type each time, in order to get a mixture of all the different nutrients.

- Eat plenty of foods rich in starch and fibre. These include bread, cereals, sweet potatoes, cornmeal, maize, millet, noodles, pasta, and rice. They are the main sources of starch and fibre, but they also provide other nutrients as well. Many people believe that these foods are fattening, which is not true. It is how we cook or serve them that adds on the calories. For example, a slice of bread with a scraping of butter on the top has twice as many calories as a slice of bread on its own.
- Eat plenty of fresh fruits and vegetables. Try to eat five servings a day. This is not as difficult as it may first appear. The five servings include *both* fruits and vegetables, not five servings of each.

fruits & vegetables

When you think about a good, healthy day's diet, it becomes clear just how easy this is to achieve. For example, for breakfast, drink a fruit smoothie (whizz together a banana, handful of strawberries and milk to taste) or have a selection of fresh fruits, chopped up and served on cereal. For lunch, enjoy a mixed crunchy salad with a yoghurt dressing served on a jacket potato. Make sure supper includes some vegetables, whether it is a quick stir-fry or a few steamed green vegetables to go with fish. Don't forget a few pieces of fruit to munch on during the day as quick snacks.

cut down on fats

Don't eat too many foods that contain a lot of fat. We all need a small amount of fat in our diets, as it is essential for health, but we need to eat more of the right sorts of fats – unsaturates – and less of the saturates such as butter, lard, and cakes. Use vegetable or nut oils for cooking and dressings and eat oily fish twice a week to provide the essential fats important for building an unborn baby's brain, eyes and nerves (*see* pages 44 for more information about fats).

Don't have sugary foods and drinks too often. Too much sugar in the diet can contribute to an excess energy intake, which can lead to obesity. Avoid cakes, biscuits, pastries, jams, marmalades, and syrups as much as possible. Instead, add sweetness to foods with ingredients such as dried and fresh fruits.

raw foods

Raw food – for example, fresh fruits, vegetables, nuts, and sprouted seeds – are great nutrient-dense foods. As cooking these foods destroys some of their nutritive value, it is a good idea to incorporate raw foods into your daily diet.

Another advantage of eating foods in their raw state is that they contain more water raw than when they are cooked. In contrast to water obtained from the tap or from bottles, the water in raw foods contains much-needed nutrients such as vitamins, proteins, electrolytes, amino acids, carbohydrates, and fatty acids. Water also increases cell metabolism and helps boost energy levels. It is possible that food sensitivities and digestive disturbances may be reduced by eating raw foods.

Eating foods in such a natural state may calm the digestive system. It is no coincidence that diets rich in natural, non-processed, or unrefined foods have also been linked to longevity.

It is very easy to include raw foods in the diet by making small changes to the way you eat. For example, pack salad ingredients into sandwiches, sprinkle nuts and seeds over salads, and enjoy more fresh fruits by whizzing them together in a food processor to make a smoothie.

When it is not possible to use raw foods, use fast methods of cooking such as steaming and stir-frying.

It is possible that food sensitivities and digestive disturbances may be reduced by eating raw foods. Eating foods in such a natural state may calm the digestive system.

Phytochemicals have been shown to help protect against cancer and heart disease. Since the body cannot store them, it is a good idea to eat as many fresh fruits and vegetables as possible.

phytochemicals

Research continues to provide reasons for eating more raw fruit and vegetables. The most recently discovered natural plant substances are known as "phytochemicals", "phyto" meaning "plant" in Greek. Phytochemicals are compounds found in food that interact in complex, complementary ways.

Phytochemicals are given weird and wonderful names that you may well come across on ingredient labels and in health magazines. Of the known health-enhancing phytochemicals, better-known examples include bioflavonoids, plant sterols, chlorophyll, and phenols.

These substances can have a major impact on your life. Certain phytochemicals have been shown to help protect against cancer and heart disease. Since the body cannot store phytochemicals, it is a good idea to eat as many fresh fruits and vegetables as possible – aiming for the recommended five portions (combined) of fresh fruits and vegetables a day to reap the full benefits that these substances provide.

Recent research comparing the effectiveness of taking supplements versus naturally occurring foods indicates that the body is able to make better use of naturally occurring foods. This is quite possibly due to the complex set of chemical reactions that occur among all the enzymes, vitamins, minerals, amino acids, and phytochemicals. Put simply, raw, organic food is the most natural and beneficial way of getting nutrients and vitamins into the body.

organic foods

"Organic" refers not to the food itself, but to how it is produced. Organic is a legal term, and all organic food production and processing is governed by strict guidelines.

The British Soil Association states that organic farming is a "safe, sustainable farming system producing healthy crops and livestock without damage to the environment".

Eating organic foods can help limit your intake of toxins such as pesticide residues and additives that could be passed on to your unborn baby. The negative cumulative effects of these substances on humans are not yet known. However, many experts believe that babies are more at risk from these toxins than adults, especially during the first few weeks of life inside the womb, when their tiny vital organs and limbs are still developing.

Some advantages of eating organic foods before and during pregnancy include the following.

● They are free from genetically modified organisms.
● Nearly all organic foods are free from pesticide residues.
● They do not contain artificial additives such as chemical sweeteners or emulsifiers and "E- numbers"; however, be aware that they may contain natural added ingredients such as sugars, salts, thickening agents, etc.
● Organic meat is free from growth promoters or hormones and contains very few, if any, antibiotics. In non-organic dairy foods, by comparison, excessive levels of antibiotics have been found. It is thought that these may cause the development of resistant strains of bacteria in babies and young children.
● Organic meat has never been reported as having a single case of BSE (mad cow disease).
● Some evidence suggests that organic foods may be richer in nutrients than their non-organic equivalents, although this is still being researched. Organic farmers use traditional methods of farming such as crop rotation and green manure to ensure that his soil is given the chance to replace

Eating organic foods can help limit your intake of toxins such as pesticide residues and additives that could be passed on to your unborn baby.

nutrients taken by the previous crops, so the argument does seem valid. Also, organic fruit and vegetables are not waxed to prolong shelf life; hence their skins – often a good source of nutrients – are safe to eat.

• The flavour of organic foods tends to be better than their non-organic equivalents. This is due partly to the fact that organic foods tend to be picked when fully ripe. Also, unlike conventionally grown fruits and vegetables, they are not fed with artificial fertilizers which encourage the plants to take up more water, resulting in a more "diluted" taste.

In the UK, farms wishing to market organic products are inspected by various bodies which have been approved by the UK Register of Organic Food Standards to check that high standards are being maintained. Producers and farmers are subject to rigid testing, including soil testing, before certification is granted; 70 to 80 percent of approved producers are certified by the Soil Association. It takes a minimum of two years for a farm to gain organic status. During this time, the farm needs to develop the soil's natural fertility and allow pesticide residues to diminish.

For these and many other reasons, aim to include as much organic food as possible in your diet.

The flavour of organic foods tends to be better than their non-organic equivalents. This is due partly to the fact that organic foods tend to be picked when fully ripe.

pregnancy nutrition

If individuals consume the RNI of a nutrient, they are very unlikely to be deficient in that nutrient.

This section includes information about the different nutrients found in your diet. As a guide, 50 percent of your daily calorie intake should come from carbohydrates; 33 to 35 percent from all fats, including a maximum 10 percent of saturated fats; and 12 percent from protein.

The recommended quantities of all nutrients for pregnant women are given by the UK's Department of Health (DOH) as reference nutrient intakes, or "RNIs".

reference nutrient intake (RNI)

Defined by the UK's DOH as an amount of a nutrient that is enough for over 97 percent of people, even those with high needs for the nutrient. Consequently, the RNI is a higher amount of a nutrient than most people need. According to the DOH, "If individuals consume the RNI of a nutrient, they are very unlikely to be deficient in that nutrient."

nutritional units of measurement

g	gram	
mg	milligram	one thousandth of 1 g
mcg	microgram	one-millionth of 1 g
ng	nanogram	one-thousand-million of 1 g
kg	kilogram	1,000 g
kcal	kilocalorie	1 calorie (unit used to measure the energy value of food)

energy

The amount of energy you have is partly dependent on the foods you eat. Your diet needs to feature plenty of good fats, carbohydrates and protein – the building blocks of energy. However, you need to limit your intake of processed foods, which may contain relatively high amounts of bad fats and sugars but very little else.

Energy is measured in calories (cals) or kilocalories (kcals).

why you need energy during pregnancy

Energy is required to both support the growth of the foetus and to enable fat to be deposited in women's bodies for use when they are breastfeeding.

how much you need

Individual calorie requirements vary enormously. Energy requirements are determined largely by the amount of energy you use, your basal metabolic rate (the rate at which your body uses energy while at complete rest), and any special needs, for example, pregnancy and breastfeeding.

Energy needed to maintain your basal metabolic rate includes energy to maintain body temperature and other normal functions such as heartbeat and breathing. If your energy intake from food is greater than your total energy use, the balance will be turned into fat and stored as an energy reserve.

Energy is needed during pregnancy to support the growing foetus and to enable fat to be deposited in the mother's body, ready for lactation. However reductions occur in physical activity and metabolic rate which help compensate for increased needs.

Consequently, the need to increase energy intakes during pregnancy is limited to a small amount during the last trimester only. The increase in estimated average requirement* (EAR) above pre-pregnancy intake is 200 kcal a day for the final three months only (weeks 27 to 40). However, women who are underweight at the beginning of pregnancy may need to eat more.

where you get it

Good sources of energy include vegetables, fruit, cereals, meat, fish, and dairy products, which supply energy as well as essential nutrients. Poor sources include highly processed foods such as cakes, pastries, and chocolate, which can contain high amounts of hidden sugar and fat and often few or no essential nutrients. These provide "empty" calories. Having sufficient calories is important, but these calories need to come from the good sources.

* Estimated Average Requirement

The EARs* for energy from the British Department of Health

15- to 18-year-old females	2,110 kcal/day
19- to 49-year-old females	1,940 kcal/day
50- to 59-year-old females	1,900 kcal/day

There are two types of carbohydrates: simple (sugars) and complex (starches and fibres). They are the body's primary source of energy. Carbohydrates should account for two-thirds of the calories you consume.

Simple carbohydrates, found in foods such as sweets and chocolate, are high in calories and provide instant energy. When you eat sugar, your blood-sugar level rises, causing your body to release insulin into the bloodstream to stabilize this raised level. It is important to keep blood-sugar levels balanced in order to maintain energy levels.

When blood sugar is low, you may feel hungry, tired, depressed, or lack concentration. When it is high – after a sugary snack – the release of insulin triggers a rapid drop in blood sugar, which makes you feel tired and hungry again. When there are high levels of sugar in the blood, the body converts the excess (in the short term) to glycogen, or to fat for long-term energy storage.

> It is important to keep blood-sugar levels balanced in order to maintain energy levels.

carbohydrates

source	carbohydrates/100g	starch/100g	sugar/100g
Wholemeal bread	41.6 g	39.8 g	1.8 g
Potatoes	17.2 g	16.6 g	0.6 g
Brown rice	81.3 g	80.0 g	1.3 g
White rice	85.8 g	85.8 g	trace
Bananas	23.2 g	2.3 g	20.9 g
Chickpeas, canned	16.1 g	15.1 g	0.4 g
Puffed wheat	67.3 g	67.0 g	0.3 g

High levels of insulin inhibit the breakdown of fat. Diabetes develops when the body cannot produce enough insulin to regulate blood sugar. This leads to a high blood-sugar level and not enough glucose going to other organs in the body.

Complex carbohydrates (starches and fibres) are found in foods such as grains, rice, potatoes, and vegetables. Our bodies have to work hard to digest starches – even harder if they are unrefined, such as wholemeal bread, pasta, and brown rice. This slows down our metabolisms, provides long-lasting energy, and helps to keep blood-sugar levels constant.

The energy in food is measured in calories. Carbohydrates provide nearly four calories per gram.

Most of your extra calories during the last three months of pregnancy should come from carbohydrates.

why you need carbohydrate during pregnancy

Carbohydrates help to provide the foetus with the supply of energy it needs for growth. Most of our extra calories during the last three months of pregnancy should come from carbohydrates.

how much you need

The requirement for carbohydrates is not affected by pregnancy. However, to maintain good health, you should eat more unrefined or "complex" carbohydrates, which means more starchy and high-fibre foods. You should also have less sugar and fewer high-sugar foods.

where to get it

Good sources of carbohydrates include grains, rice, bread, fruits, and vegetables. Poor sources of carbohydrates include processed foods such as biscuits, pastries, and chocolate.

fat

Essential fatty acids are vital for the brain and nervous system, cardiovascular system, and skin.

Fats and oils are made up of molecules of fatty acids and glycerol. All fats are made up of a combination of three types of fatty acid. A fat is said to be saturated, mono-unsaturated, or poly-unsaturated, depending on which type of fatty acid is present in largest proportion. Saturated fats such as butter, are solid at room temperature. Mono-saturated fats, like olive oil, are liquid at room temperature. Polyunsaturated fats, such as sunflower oil, are liquid at room temperature and they also remain liquid even when it is cold.

Some fatty acids in the diet are absolutely essential to health. These essential fatty acids, or EFAs, are found in plant and fish oils, e.g. linoleic acid and linolenic acid. Essential fatty acids cannot be made in the body, so, like vitamins and minerals, they need to be eaten in the diet.

Fats are much higher in calories than either protein or carbohydrate. There are nine kilocalories (kcal) in every gram of fat, compared to four per gram of protein, or 3.75 per gram of carbohydrates.

why you need fat during pregnancy

Some fat is essential in everyone's diet. Foods that contain fats provide a concentrated source of energy, and the fat-soluble vitamins A, D, E, and K. These vitamins are vital for normal growth and development.

Essential fatty acids are vital for the brain and nervous system, immune system, cardiovascular system, and skin; hence, they are necessary during pregnancy to help ensure the proper development of the baby.

Essential fats have also been found to be crucial for development of the baby's brain, eyes, and central nervous system (*Ref. 2.1*). A good supply can help to prevent low birth weights and decrease the likelihood of a premature birth with all its potential risks, including cerebral palsy, blindness, deafness, etc. (*Ref. 2.2*).

how much you need

Unlike most other nutrients, there is no requirement, as such, for fats. However, the British Nutrition Foundation Task Force and the World Health Organization have recommended that women planning pregnancy, and those already pregnant, should have an adequate intake of essential fatty acids. Most authorities now agree that fat should constitute about 35 percent of the energy content of your diet, with no more than 10 percent coming from animal sources.

An optimum amount of essential fatty acids required for pregnancy is not known. But it is thought that, on the whole, most people living in Britain already get sufficient to satisfy their needs. However, recent surveys have shown that many people's diets are low in linoleic acid, one of the important essential fats (see right).

where to get it

Saturated fats come mainly from animal products such as butter, lard, suet, dripping, meat, eggs, full-fat milk, cheese, and full-fat yoghurt. Saturated fats are also found in hard margarines (hydrogenated vegetable oil), which contain trans-fatty acids (*see* below). Also high in saturated fats are coconut oil and palm oil.

Unsaturated fats are generally liquid at room temperature and come from vegetable sources, particularly oils, e.g. olive, sunflower, soya, peanut, and sesame. Linolenic acid and linoleic acid are also found in oils, e.g sesame, safflower, soya, and maize oil, as well as in nuts, seeds, fatty fish (herring, mackerel, sardines, and salmon), and soya drinks.

Margarines and low-fat spreads often contain hydrogenated vegetable oil. Hydrogenation involves transforming the vegetable oil into a solid fat by changing its chemical structure (it becomes a trans-fatty acid). It was once thought that all vegetable fats, solid or liquid, had fewer detrimental health effects than animal fats. However, research indicates that trans-fatty acids can cause free-radical damage – linked with heart disease and cancer – within the body's cells. Now some soft margarines have the trans-fatty acids removed.

In preference to hard margarine, use olive oil or a small amount of butter.

During pregnancy, protein is required not only for the growth of the baby, but also for the growth of other protein-rich tissues.

Protein consists of building blocks called amino acids. There are two types of amino acids: essential and non-essential. Essential amino acids must be obtained directly from food, while the body can produce non-essential amino acids from other sources. You therefore need to make sure that your diet contains enough essential amino acids.

why you need protein during pregnancy

Protein is needed to help the body build or repair muscles, tissues, hair, and organs, and to maintain an effective immune and hormonal system. During pregnancy, protein is required not only for the growth of the baby, but also for the growth of other protein-rich tissues, including extra blood cells, the uterus in particular, and the placenta.

Proteins in the diet are broken down by digestive enzymes and absorbed into the blood as amino acids. These are then taken to build and repair cells and carry out their other roles, as required. Any extra protein may be used for energy or stored as fat. During pregnancy, protein is used efficiently: less protein is used for energy and more is stored for use by the baby.

protein

protein source	protein intake/source
600 ml semi-skimmed milk	19.80 g
175 g salmon fillet, steamed	35.18 g
225 g sirloin steak (lean and fat), raw	37.35 g
225 g tofu (soya bean curd), steamed	18.23 g
50 g Cheddar cheese	12.75 g
250 g green or brown lentils, boiled in salted water	22.00 g
225 g white rice, boiled	6.00 g

how much you need

The RNI for protein is 54 g. This increases by 11 percent for pregnant women, or six grams per day. However, some nutritionists consider this estimate to be too high. The overall need for protein depends on both the quality of the protein, and the dietary intake of vitamins and minerals. This determines how efficiently you use protein. In other words, if you eat good-quality protein and are not vitamin and mineral deficient, you can afford to eat less than this. The minimum requirement for protein during pregnancy is 49 g per day.

where to get it

The best-quality protein foods (in terms of their amino acid balance) include eggs, soya beans, meat, fish, dairy products, and poultry. Vegetarian protein foods, e.g. pulses, grains, nuts, seeds, and manufactured vegetable protein foods, don't contain all the essential amino acids, but if eaten in combination – pulses with grains, pulses with nuts, or nuts with seeds – they can meet the body's daily protein needs.

For example, good protein-providing vegetarian meals include lentil soup with wholemeal bread, vegetable kebabs with nut sauces, and vegetable and cheese omelettes.

Unborn babies cannot make protein, so if mothers do not eat enough, they have to go without.

The following excellent-quality protein foods all provide 20 g of protein: 400 g brown rice, 84 g canned tuna, 100 g sardines, two medium eggs, 450 g yoghurt, and 275 g tofu (soya-bean curd).

Unborn babies cannot make protein, so if mothers do not eat enough, they have to go without.

daily requirement of protein

	age	15-18	19-50
normal daily requirement		45 g	45 g
during pregnancy		51 g	51 g
during lactation up to 4 mths		56 g	56 g
during lactation, 4 mths +		53 g	53 g

Minerals are essential for almost every bodily process. For example, oxygen is carried in the blood by an iron compound; a lack of this mineral can lead to anaemia. Calcium, magnesium, and phosphorus help make up bones and teeth.

Magnesium, calcium, and zinc, are important both before and during pregnancy. Research has shown that there is no increased need for other minerals during pregnancy. In addition, normal intakes in the UK are generally well above the recommended intake, so there is very little likelihood of anyone in the UK being deficient in them. Such minerals include sodium chloride, potassium, copper, iodine, selenium, manganese, fluoride, chromium, nickel, and silicon.

Ninety-nine percent of the body's calcium content is found in bones and teeth, with one percent in blood plasma and soft tissues. The major part of phosphorus in the body is associated with calcium in the bones.

why you need calcium during pregnancy

Calcium is crucial for the formation of both healthy teeth and bones in an unborn baby.

> Calcium, magnesium, and phosphorus help make up bones and teeth.

calcium & phosphorus

calcium source	calcium intake/source
600 ml semi-skimmed milk	680 mg
40 g (2 tbsp) almonds	96 mg
50 g Cheddar cheese	360 mg
45 g (3) dried figs	112.5 mg
20 g (1 tbsp) sesame seeds	134 mg
100 g (individual pot) Greek yoghurt	200 mg
50 g sardines canned in oil	275 mg

phosphorus source	phosphorus intake/source
600 ml semi-skimmed milk	540 mg
40 g (2 tbsp) almonds	220 mg
50 g Cheddar cheese	245 mg
45 g (3) dried figs	40 mg
20 g (1 tbsp) sesame seeds	144 mg
100 g (individual pot) Greek yoghurt	170 mg
50 g sardines canned in oil	260 mg

how much calcium you need

The RNI for women is 800 mg for 15- to 18-year-old females and 700 mg for females over 19 years of age. The average intake of women in the UK aged 16 to 34 is 689 mg per day. This means that a number of women have less than the recommended intake.

During pregnancy, calcium absorption increases, but no additional calcium is generally needed. One exception is the pregnant adolescent, whose bone mineralization (hardening) may still be taking place. Consequently, the needs for dietary calcium both for herself and for the developing baby are particularly high.

Calcium concentrations are higher in a developing foetus than in its mother, which suggests that your baby will maintain an adequate supply at your expense.

how much phosphorus you need

The RNI for 19 years and over is 550 mg per day. Lactating women need an extra 440 mg per day, totalling 990 mg per day.

where to get calcium & phosphorus

Both are found in the following foods. Almost half our calcium is obtained from milk and cheese, and a quarter comes from bread and other cereals. Just 600 ml of milk daily will provide a bit under the recommended intake. Other good sources include yoghurt, tofu and soya drinks enriched with calcium, canned fish (where the bones are eaten) such as sardines and salmon, dark-green, leafy vegetables, dried fruit, nuts, and seeds, especially sesame seeds.

It is vital to include other trace minerals and vitamins, such as vitamin D, in the diet to make sure that calcium is absorbed and used by the body. Alcohol and caffeine can inhibit its absorption.

Vegans should pay particular attention to their calcium intakes to ensure adequate levels.

daily requirement of phosphorus

age 19+

normal/pregnancy	**550 mg**
during lactation	**990 mg**

zinc

Helping to maintain a healthy immune system and assisting in cell replication are just some of the functions of zinc.

Vitamins A, E, and B$_6$ as well as magnesium, calcium, and phosphorus all help the body to absorb zinc. Stress, alcohol, and a low-protein intake can prevent it from being absorbed. If we become deficient in zinc, we may experience acne or greasy skin, loss of appetite, and maybe depression.

why you need zinc during pregnancy

Zinc is involved in the process of cell replication. It is therefore important to have a good supply in the early stages of pregnancy.

A number of studies have found that women with low zinc levels had a greater tendency to have babies with congenital malformations of the central nervous system (*Ref. 2.3*). Low intakes early in pregnancy have been related to growth retardation and lower birth weights (*Ref 2.4*). See "Zinc" pages 16–7.

how much you need

Extra zinc is required during pregnancy, but women have the ability to absorb this mineral more efficiently during pregnancy. Therefore, the dietary requirement for zinc in pregnancy is the same as for non-pregnant women: seven milligrams per day.

Long-term use of contraceptive pills may inhibit the absorption of zinc and cause the body to excrete more. Evidence of this is slight, but it is still recommended that women should make a real effort to eat a healthy diet with foods that contain zinc if they have just come off the pill.

where to get it

Sources include red meat, shellfish, – mussels, crab, and lobster – canned sardines, turkey, Parmesan and other hard or crumbly cheeses (Cheddar and Cheshire), nuts and seeds (including peanut butter and tahini), wholegrain cereals, pulses (dried peas, beans, and lentils), green vegetables such as watercress and spinach, and dried apricots, figs and raisins.

zinc source	zinc intake/source
200 g roast beef	13.60 mg
20 g anchovies, canned	0.64 mg
285 g stewing lamb	19.70 mg
20 g (1 tbsp) pine nuts	1.30 mg
50 g green lentils	1.95 mg
200 g crab meat (½ crab)	11.00 mg
225 g stewing steak	19.60 mg

iron

Iron is needed for healthy blood and muscles, and is vital for cell respiration – the process by which cells generate energy. Lack of iron in the body leads to a common form of anaemia.

why you need iron during pregnancy

About 40 percent of women aged 18 to 34 have low blood iron stores. Menstrual losses account for the fact that a woman's iron needs are much greater than the iron needs of a man.

During pregnancy, the placenta can deliver large quantities of iron to the baby, even if doing so means depriving its mother of iron. If women are suffering from iron deficiency, it is often a result of poor nutrition.

how much you need

The RNI for 19- to 50-year-old women is 14.8 mg per day. The average intake among women in the UK is 10.5 mg per day, so there are many women who are not reaching the target. Therefore it is important to try to achieve the recommended iron intake before becoming pregnant, to help prevent a deficiency during the pregnancy.

Requirements for iron are not increased during pregnancy. This is partly because there is no loss of iron through menstruation, and also because iron is absorbed more efficiently during pregnancy.

where to get it

The two sources of iron in the diet are haeme iron from animal protein and non-haeme iron from plant sources. The body finds it easier to absorb haeme iron. We are capable of absorbing 20 to 40 percent of the iron from meat and only five to 20 percent available from vegetable sources. Consequently, women need to eat a lot more of the non-haeme sources to obtain a good supply of iron.

Good sources of haeme iron include meat; moderate sources include lean meat, chicken, and fish; and small amounts are found in milk.

Good sources of non-haeme iron include cereals fortified with iron, wholegrain bread, dark-green, leafy vegetables (such as watercress, spinach, broccoli, and Savoy cabbage), nuts, pulses seeds, figs, apricots, prunes, raisins, liquorice, and plain chocolate. Vitamin C and folic acid aid in the absorption of iron, so it is advisable to eat good sources of these nutrients at the same time. Try to include good sources of these vitamins in the same meal as your iron source.

iron source	iron intake/source
110 g spinach, raw	2.31 mg
20 g (1 tbsp) sesame seeds	2.08 mg
20 g (1 tbsp) tahini paste	2.12 mg
45 g (3) dried figs	1.89 mg
225 g rump steak, grilled	7.90 mg
60 g (medium bowl) Special K®	7.98 mg
20 g (1 tbsp) oat or wheat bran	9.0 mg

magnesium

Magnesium is vital for the release of energy, building strong bones, teeth, and muscles, and regulating body temperature. It also helps the body absorb and metabolize other nutrients such as calcium and vitamin C.

why you need magnesium during pregnancy

Magnesium was the mineral most closely associated with birth weight in one study, which found that premature birth and the risk of low birth weight was increased with low intakes early in pregnancy (*Ref. 2.5*).

how much you need

The RNI for women, pregnant or otherwise, is 270 mg per day. The average female intake is 237 mg, so some women need to increase their dietary intake prior to conception.

The good news is that absorption of magnesium increases during pregnancy. By contrast, when women are breastfeeding, they need an extra 50 mg a day.

where to get it

Excellent sources of magnesium include wholegrain cereal products such as. wholemeal and granary bread, wholewheat pasta,and brown rice; nuts, e.g. almonds and cashew nuts; seeds; pulses; green, leafy vegetables such as spinach; peas; sweetcorn; courgettes; parsnips; milk; yoghurt; lean meat; dried figs; apricots; raisins; and bananas.

magnesium source	magnesium intake/source
30 g (2 slices) wholemeal bread	60.8 mg
55 g brown rice	60.5 mg
20 g (1 tbsp) sunflower seeds	78.0 mg
40 g (2 tbsp) Brazil nuts	164.0 mg
20 g (4) rye crispbread	20.0 mg
45 g (3) dried figs	36.0 mg
20 g (1 tbsp) wheat bran	104.0 mg

vitamins

Vitamins "turn-on" enzymes, which help to make all body processes happen. We need vitamins for a variety of functions; these include producing energy, balancing hormones, boosting the immune system, and making healthy skin. There are 13 essential vitamins in total, each with a special role to play. These can be divided into two groups: fat-soluble (A, D, E, and K) and water-soluble (C and B-complex). Water-soluble vitamins cannot be stored by the body, so foods containing these should be eaten daily. They can also be destroyed by overcooking, especially boiling vegetables or fruit in lots of water. It is best to eat fresh fruit and vegetables raw or lightly cooked.

Both B and C vitamins are necessary for turning food into energy. In addition, vitamins A, C, and E are all antioxidants, which help protect against cancer, heart disease, and pollution. Vitamin D also helps to control the body's calcium intake.

B VITAMINS

B-complex vitamins cover a large group of substances, including B_1 (thiamin), B_2 (riboflavin), B_3 (niacin), folic acid, B_5 (pantothenic acid), B_6 (pyridoxine), and B_{12} (cyanocobalamine). These vitamins play many roles including metabolizing food and converting it into energy, assisting in the production of red blood cells, and aiding the development and maintenance of a healthy nervous system.

B_1 thiamin

This vitamin helps the body to convert both protein and carbohydrate into energy. Vitamin B_1 is also used in brain function, and metabolism. Tiredness, weakness, and mood swings are classic symptoms of a vitamin B_1 deficiency.

why you need vitamin B_1 during pregnancy
Low intakes, of thiamin and vitamin B_3 (niacin), have been associated with lower birth weights.

In one study, mothers who had a low intake of thiamine and niacin had a nine-fold higher probability of having a low birth weight baby compared to the mothers who had high intakes. The same picture emerged with several other B vitamins, including riboflavin and vitamin B_6 (Ref. 2.6).

how much you need
The RNI for non-pregnant women is 0.8 mg per day. This amount should also be sufficient to cover pregnancy needs until the third trimester, when, due to increased energy requirements, the intake of thiamine should increase to 0.9 mg.

Other B vitamins assist in the absorption of thiamine. Tea, coffee, alcohol, cooking, and refined foods can all restrict thiamine absorption.

where to get it
Good sources include wholegrain or enriched breads; breakfast cereals; Quorn®; pulses (peas, beans, and lentils); brewer's yeast; peanut butter; wheat germ, green vegetables such as cabbage, Brussels sprouts, asparagus, and watercress; peppers; and tomatoes.

vitamin B_1 source	vitamin B_1 intake/source
20 g tahini paste	0.19 mg
20 g (1 tbsp) sesame seeds	0.19 mg
20 g (1 tbsp) sunflower seeds	0.32 mg
50 g peanuts	0.57 mg
100 g Quorn®	36.60 mg
200 g baked potatoes	0.74 mg
200 g pork loin	1.76 mg

B$_2$ riboflavin

Vitamin B$_2$, or riboflavin, plays an essential role in the release of energy from proteins, fats, and carbohydrates.

why you need riboflavin during pregnancy

Riboflavin requirements relate to protein requirements. An increase in protein requirements during pregnancy means an increased need for riboflavin.

how much you need

The RNI for women is 1.1 mg, increasing to 1.4 mg during pregnancy. The average intake in the UK is 1.57 mg per day. However, research indicates that the intakes of some women, particularly those who are slimming, tend to be lower than the RNI. Make sure you are eating good sources of riboflavin both before and during pregnancy.

where to get it

Excellent sources include milk and milk products. Six hundred millilitres of milk provides all the riboflavin you need in a day. Other good sources include cereal products, wheat germ, meat and meat products, yoghurt, cheese, eggs, pilchards, soya products, brewer's yeast and yeast extracts, and green, leafy vegetables.

B$_3$ niacin

Vitamin B$_3$, or niacin works with thiamin and riboflavin in releasing energy from food.

why you need niacin during pregnancy

Niacin is essential for cell division, normal growth, healthy skin, brain and nerve function, the tongue, and digestive organs.

how much you need

The RNI for non-pregnant women is 13 mg. Niacin requirements, like thiamin and riboflavin, are related to energy intake.

where to get it

Good sources include meat and meat products, wholegrain cereals and bread, oily fish, poultry, eggs, cheese, brewer's yeast and yeast extracts, pulses (peas, beans, and lentils), dried fruit, and nuts.

vitamin B$_2$ source	vitamin B$_2$ intake/source
40 g (2 tbsp) almonds	0.30 mg
100 g (4) passion-fruit	12.00 mg
30 g (handful) mushrooms	0.25 mg
50 g sardines	0.18 mg
200 g duck, roasted	0.94 mg
50 g Cheddar cheese	0.20 mg

vitamin B$_3$ source	vitamin B$_3$ intake/source
50 g peanuts	6.90 mg
30 g (handful) mushrooms	2.56 mg
50 g smoked salmon	4.4 mg
65 g (½ small can) tuna in brine	9.36 mg
110 g chicken meat	11.30 mg
60 g (medium bowl) Special K®	12.00 mg
20 g (1 tbsp) wheat bran	5.92 mg

B$_6$ pyridoxine

Vitamin B$_6$ is needed for growth, to convert protein into energy, protect against heart disease, regulate the menstrual cycle, and help with the functioning of the nervous and immune systems. B$_6$ supplementation can also help relieve premenstrual tension.

why you need vitamin B$_6$ during pregnancy

Vitamin B$_6$ and folic acid are frequently associated with pregnancy complications and adverse outcomes (*Ref. 2.7*). Vitamin B$_6$ is essential for breaking down protein for use in the growth of new body tissues and the production of antibodies and red blood cells.

how much you need

Vitamin B6 requirements are related to protein intake. The RNI of vitamin B$_6$ for both pregnant and non-pregnant women is 1.2 mg per day. The average intake of vitamin B$_6$ from food is 1.6 mg per day. However, there are women whose intakes are below the recommended amount (*Ref. 2.8*).

where to get it

Good sources include meat, chicken, and fish. Others include wholegrain and enriched breads, breakfast cereals, brewer's yeast, potatoes, beans, lentils, green vegetables, bananas, melons, and peanuts.

B$_{12}$ cyanocobalamine

Vitamin B$_{12}$ is linked with folic acid in having a central role in the production of red blood cells and the prevention of anaemia.

why you need vitamin B$_{12}$ during pregnancy

Vitamin B$_{12}$ assists in maintaining the metabolism and the nervous system. It also aids in the prevention of pernicious anaemia, and assists the proper formation of blood cells.

how much you need

The RNI for non-pregnant and pregnant women is 1.5 ug per day – a very small amount. The average intake is 5.4 ug, so few women are likely to be deficient.

where to get it

It is found almost exclusively in foods of animal origin, e.g sardines, pilchards, milk, cheese, and eggs. Vegans sources include Quorn®, fortified soya drinks or Marmite®.

vitamin B$_{12}$ source	vitamin B$_{12}$ intake/source
50 g sardines, canned in oil	14.00 ug
200 g duck, roasted	6.00 ug
65 g (½ small can) tuna in brine	2.80 ug
70 g cod, baked	3.40 ug
225 g beef steak	4.50 ug
20 g (2 medium) scrambled eggs	2.52 ug

vitamin B$_6$ source	vitamin B$_6$ intake/source
20 g (1 tbsp) sesame seeds	0.15 mg
40 g (2 tbsp) hazelnuts	0.24 mg
150 g (medium) banana	0.44 mg
200 g (medium) avocado	0.72 mg
200 g baked potatoes	1.08 mg
400 g (1) chicken breast	2.12 mg
60 g (medium bowl) Special K®	1.32 mg

Folic acid plays a vital role in cell division and in creating healthy blood cells. It is also needed to enable the body to absorb iron – a nutrient needed for healthy blood.

folic acid

Folic acid is important for the developing spinal cord. It helps make new cells and genetic material, and aids in the prevention of neural tube defects...

why you need folic acid during pregnancy

Folic acid is important for the unborn baby's developing spinal cord. It is needed to make new cells and genetic material, and, most importantly, aids in the prevention of neural tube defects (NTDs) such as spina bifida.

Spina bifida – a condition in which the spinal cord does not develop properly – has been strongly linked to a lack of folic acid. Folic acid is also needed to help prevent the development of certain types of anaemia and promote the growth of foetal tissues and organs. It is also needed for the formation of protein tissues in the mother and the foetus.

folic acid source	folic acid intake/source
50 g peanuts	55.0 ug
20 g (1 tbsp) sesame seeds	19.4 ug
180 g (whole) orange	55.8 ug
110 g spinach, raw	165.0 ug
100 g asparagus, boiled	155.0 ug
35 g Brussels sprouts	93.5 ug
200 g baked potatoes	88.0 ug
60 g (medium bowl) Special K®	198.0 ug
55 g brown rice	27.0 ug

how much you need

The normal RNI for adults is 200 ug. Pregnant women need an extra 100 ug per day.

The UK's Department of Health recommends that "Women who are planning to become pregnant or who may become pregnant should have a daily 400 ug folic acid supplement for at least three months before conceiving, and continue taking it for the first three months of pregnancy." (*Ref. 2.19*). The first 12 weeks are the most critical, as after this period the baby's neural tube will have passed through its most vulnerable period.

The average intake is between 109 and 203 ug per day, so eating foods rich in folic acid, as well as supplementation is essential to reach the total of 600 ug.

A survey of 23,000 women showed that those who supplemented their diet with folic acid during the first six weeks of pregnancy had a 75 percent lower incidence of NTDs than those who didn't (*Ref. 2.10*).

Genetics also play a part in NTDs – not all can be prevented by folic acid supplementation. If either parent has spina bifida, their risk of having a NTD baby is increased tenfold (*Ref. 2.11*). If there is a known case of a NTD, most commonly spina bifida, in either family, it is important to discuss this with your doctor before pregnancy.

where to get it

Folic acid occurs naturally in many foods, particularly plant foliage. Good sources include green, leafy vegetables – Savoy cabbage, spring greens, Brussels sprouts and spinach – broccoli, asparagus, wholemeal bread and cereal, dark-yellow vegetables and fruit – oranges, grapefruit, mangoes, papaya, peaches, and pumpkin – beans, enriched grain products, and nuts.

Try to eat much of your fresh vegetables and fruits raw, steamed, microwaved or quickly stir-fried – folic acid is destroyed by heat and leaks out into cooking water.

It is quite a challenge to achieve 600 ug of folic acid through diet alone, so it is advisable to take a recommended supplement.

daily requirement of folic acid

▮ normal daily requirement	**200 ug**
▮ during pregnancy	**300 ug**
▮ whilst planning pregnancy	**600 ug**

One of the antioxidant vitamins, Vitamin C is needed for a variety of functions: helping to turn food into energy; strengthening the immune system; keeping bones and joints strong; growth and healthy body tissue; healing wounds; and the absorption of iron (*see page 51*). Deficiency in vitamin C can result in a lack of energy, colds, bleeding or tender gums, and slow healing of wounds.

vitamin C source	vitamin C intake/source
100 g strawberries	77.0 mg
180 g (whole) orange	97.2 mg
85 g (whole) kiwi fruit	50.2 mg
75 g guava	172.5 mg
100 g blackcurrants	200.0 mg
200 g spring greens, cooked	154.0 mg
200 g (whole medium) red pepper	280.0 mg

vitamin c

why you need vitamin C during pregnancy

Vitamin C assists the absorption of iron from plant sources. A deficiency can have a negative effect on the production of collagen – a protein needed for bone structure, cartilage, muscle, and blood vessels.

Vitamin C levels in foetal blood may be 50 percent higher than in the mother's blood. The placenta has the ability to concentrate some nutrients to the benefit of the foetus.

how much you need

The RNI for non-pregnant women is 40 mg per day, increasing to 50 mg per day for pregnant women and 70 mg per day during breastfeeding. The average intake for women in the UK is 62 mg per day, but significantly lower in 16- to 24-year-olds.

Remember that vitamin C is a water-soluble vitamin which cannot be stored by the body, so foods containing the vitamin should be eaten daily.

where to get it

Good sources include vegetables such as spring greens, cabbage, red and yellow peppers, watercress, potatoes, peas, and mange tout; fruit such as oranges, strawberries, kiwi fruit, grapefruit, and other citrus fruits, blackcurrants, mangoes, papayas, nectarines, peaches, raspberries, and tomatoes.

Vitamin C is destroyed by oxygen and heat, and it can also leach into water during cooking, so avoid overcooking its food sources.

Avoid smoking, stress, and fried foods, which prevent vitamin C from being absorbed and used by the body.

70 mg
60 mg
50 mg
40 mg
30 mg
20 mg
10 mg

daily requirement of vitamin C

■	normal daily requirement	**40 mg**
■	during pregnancy	**50 mg**
■	during lactation	**70 mg**

vitamin A retinol

Vitamin A is found in animal products; betacarotene is found in plant foods and converted by the body into vitamin A.

Vitamin A is essential for growth, healthy skin and hair, good vision, and healthy tooth enamel. Betacarotene is an important antioxidant essential for protection against heart disease and cancer, and as an immune booster. It is also needed for healthy skin and hair, and night vision.

why you need vitamin A during pregnancy

Vitamin A has antioxidant and protective properties which protect against damage to cells.

how much you need

The RNI for women is 600 ug, with an increase to 700 ug for pregnant women. The average intake for women in the UK is 1,490 ug per day.

where to get it

Vitamin A is found in animal products as retinol (pre-formed vitamin A) and in plant foods as betacarotene, which the body can convert to vitamin A.

Sources of vitamin A (retinol) include liver and liver products, e.g. pâté (but see page 70), oily fish such as herring, mackerel, and trout, fish liver oils, milk, cheese and margarine (fortified by law with vitamins A and D), and egg yolks. Foods rich in betacarotene include: carrots; dark-green, leafy vegetables such as spinach, broccoli, cabbage, kale, Brussels sprouts, and watercress; asparagus; peas; beans; courgettes; leeks; lettuce; tomatoes; sweet potatoes; pumpkins; apricots; peaches (fresh and dried); mangoes; passion-fruit; papayas; plums; watermelons; and yellow-fleshed melons. Too much vitamin A (in the form of retinol) from animal sources can build up in the liver and cause damage to the foetus. However, this is extremely rare – you would need to eat a large quantity over a long period of time for this to be a problem (see page 70 for more information about vitamin A intake). Vegetable sources of vitamin A (betacarotene) don't cause any defects in an unborn child. (Ref. 2.12).

vitamin A source	vitamin A intake/source
225 g kipper	74.25 ug
20 g (2 medium) scrambled eggs	354.00 ug
100 g (individual pot) Greek yoghurt	115.00 ug
50 g Cheddar cheese	162.50 ug
50 g (¼ pack) cream cheese	192.50 ug
600 ml semi-skimmed milk	312.40 ug

betacarotene source	betacarotene intake/source
350 g (whole) papaya	2,835 ug
225 g mangoes	4,050 ug
110 g spinach, raw	3,888 ug
200 g sweet potatoes	4,356 ug
200 g (whole medium) red pepper	7,560 ug
100 g carrot, raw and unpeeled	8,115 ug

vitamin D

Vitamin D, also known as calciferol, works with the mineral calcium. Both are essential for normal growth and for the growth and maintenance of healthy bones and teeth.

why you need vitamin D during pregnancy

Vitamin D supports foetal growth, the calcification (or the addition of calcium) of bone, and tooth and enamel formation.

how much you need

Because sufficient vitamin D is obtained from sunlight, no RNI has been set for dietary sources of vitamin D for non-pregnant women.

However, research indicates that an unborn baby may suffer rather than the mother if she becomes deficient in this vitamin. Therefore the UK government recommends an additional 10 ug a day during pregnancy. A supplement may be required to achieve that amount.

where to get it

Vitamin D is made by the skin in the presence of sunlight. If you go outside every day, you are capable of synthesizing enough vitamin D from April to October to satisfy needs during those months and to build up liver stores to last through the remainder of the year.

In addition, good food sources include seaweed; oily fish such as tuna, mackerel, kippers, canned sardines, and canned or fresh salmon; cod liver oil; liver (but *see* page 70); eggs; butter and margarine; cheese; milk or soya drinks fortified with vitamin D; yoghurt; and cereal fortified with vitamin D.

Vitamins A, C, and E help to protect vitamin D. Fried foods and a lack of sunlight work against it.

vitamin D source	vitamin D intake/source
50 g sardines, canned	3.75 ug
225 g kipper	56.25 ug
210 g (½ large can) salmon	26.25 ug
65 g (½ small can) tuna in brine	2.60 ug
120 g (2 medium) scrambled eggs	1.86 ug
50 g Cheddar cheese	0.13 ug

vitamin E

Vitamin E – an antioxidant vitamin – is needed to help develop and maintain strong cells, especially in the blood.

why you need vitamin E during pregnancy

General health requirements.

how much you need

The suggested safe intake of 3-4 mg per day is easily obtained from a well-balanced diet.

where to get it

Good sources include avocados, mangoes, tomatoes, sweet potatoes, green, leafy vegetables (spinach, watercress, and lettuce), nuts, seeds, wheat germ, wholegrain cereals, milk, egg yolks, soft margarine, vegetable oils, sardines, and salmon.

vitamin E source	vitamin E intake/source
20 g (1 tbsp) sunflower seeds	7.6 mg
40 g (2 tbsp) hazelnuts	5.0 mg
40 g (2 tbsp) almonds	4.8 mg
20 g (1 tbsp) pine nuts	2.7 mg
20 g (1 tbsp) peanuts	2.0 mg
200 g (whole medium) avocado	6.4 mg
15 ml (1 tbsp) sunflower oil	9.8 mg

supplements

In theory, if you eat a well-balanced (see pages 34–5) and healthy diet, you should not need supplements. However, the UK's Department of Health has recommended that all women who are trying to conceive or who could be pregnant should take a daily supplement of 400 ug of folic acid.

It has also suggested taking a supplement of vitamin D during pregnancy to achieve the additional intake of 10 ug a day. Any other decisions on whether to take a supplement are up to each individual.

There is no doubt that vitamin and mineral supplements have a valuable role to play, both in the prevention and treatment of a wide variety of health problems. However, pills are artificially manufactured, and there is growing evidence that naturally derived vitamins and minerals in food are more effective than those that are synthetically manufactured.

Nutrients in food are more easily absorbed by the body. It is therefore the advice of many experts that you eat a good varied diet to obtain all the essential nutrients you need from your food.

pregnancy & food safety

foods & safety

The immune system does not function as well as usual during pregnancy, so women are far more susceptible to the germs responsible for food poisoning.

safety in the home

Taking care in preparing food is very important if you are to avoid food poisoning. This is highly advisable, particularly during the first stages of pregnancy, because the immune system of an unborn baby is not sufficiently well-developed to fight infection.

general tips on food safety

- Wash your hands before and after handling food, especially when touching raw or cooked poultry and meat.
- Keep food surfaces in the kitchen clean and keep pets away from all food preparation areas.
- Use separate boards for preparing raw and cooked poultry and meat.
- Wash all boards thoroughly after using them.
- Don't eat food that has gone past its "use-by" date.
- Cook all food thoroughly, especially eggs, poultry, and meat.
- When reheating food, make sure it is piping hot all the way through.
- Wash all fruit and vegetables.
- Store eggs away from other foods as their shells may carry harmful bacteria. Also wash your hands after handling eggs.

fridge

- Keep your fridge between 0° and 4°C.
- Keep raw food on the bottom shelf of the fridge, so that if for any reason it leaks, it will not drip onto other foods. Keep raw food away from any cooked food.
- Wrap raw poultry and meat well, to prevent them from dripping or leaking onto other foods.

pets

- Pets and other animals can pass on harmful bacteria that may be present in their faeces. If these bacteria or other organisms are passed into your mouth, you can become infected with the bacteria, so after handling pets and animals it is important not to touch your mouths and to wash your hands before eating or preparing food.
- Cat litter trays need to be kept clean. If you have to clean them always wear rubber gloves, and wash your gloved hands, then your bare hands, thoroughly afterwards.
- Also wear rubber gloves when gardening to protect your hands from toxoplasma, which may be present in the garden soil. Washing your hands after gardening is also prudent even if you have worn gloves.
- Sheep may miscarry or give birth to sick lambs following an infection, so don't help with lambing, handle newborn lambs, or come into close contact with sheep that have just given birth or miscarried. Boots and clothing that may be contaminated should not be brought into the house, but they should be cleaned thoroughly by someone else outside the farmhouse.

A blood test can determine whether or not you have listeriosis. Contact the doctor if symptoms develop (see below). A course of antibiotics can often prevent foetal infections.

safety in the diet

It is suspected that the immune system may not function as well as usual during pregnancy so women may be more susceptible to the germs responsible for food poisoning. Infections caused by contact with infected food or animals include the following.

listeria

Listeria bacteria can cause an illness known as listeriosis. This can feel like mild flu, with aches and pains, sore throat, and high temperatures. In rare circumstances it can progress into a more serious condition, causing septicaemia (blood poisoning) and meningitis in newborn babies.

However, in some people the symptoms are so slight that they may not even be aware that they have had the illness. During pregnancy, listeria can be a problem since it can be passed from a mother to her unborn baby.

Although infection is rare, it is obviously sensible to avoid foods that are major sources of the listeria bacteria (see the rest of this chapter for more information) both before and during pregnancy.

Pregnant women are 20 times more likely than other healthy adults to get listeriosis.

Symptoms of infection can develop from two to 30 days after eating contaminated food.

Salmonella is one of the most common causes of food poisoning. It rarely causes damage to an unborn baby... but it is best to avoid any stress to your unborn child.

salmonella

Salmonella is one of the most common causes of food poisoning. It rarely causes damage to an unborn baby since the bacterium does not normally cross the placenta, but it is best to avoid salmonella to maintain good health and avoid any stress to your unborn child. Symptoms of this food poisoning include vomiting, diarrhoea, very high temperatures, and dehydration. If you have salmonella, drink lots of fluids to replace lost liquids.

toxoplasmosis

This infection is caused by a parasite. It is not usually dangerous and may even go unnoticed in the healthy adult or unborn baby with just flu-like symptoms. However, in rare incidences toxoplasmosis has affected the health of the mother and/or the baby.

According to the Tommy's Campaign (see "Useful Addresses", page 143), three out of 10 people will have been infected by the age of 30. If you have had toxoplasmosis, you will be immune for life – a blood test can identify whether or not you are immune. If concerned, ask the GP for such a test before you become pregnant.

The most common source of the bacteria may be found in animal's faeces, specifically that of cats. Sensible hygiene precautions should be followed. Eating raw or uncooked meat or contact with infected soil can also pass on the disease.

cheese

what to avoid

The following cheeses can carry potentially dangerous bacteria called *Listeria monocytogenes*, although cases of listeria infection are rare.

Avoid all soft, semi-soft, and blue cheeses. To be more specific, it is best to avoid both pasteurized and unpasteurized soft cheeses which usually have a surface mould and edible rind – for example, Brie, Camembert, feta, Montrachet, Neufchâtel, and Pont l'Evêque.

It is also best to avoid slightly more solid cheeses that do not grate easily and that are often coated with wax to preserve moisture and extend shelf-life, such as Asiago, Belle Passe, Havarti, Muenster, Port-Salut, and Taleggio. Also stay away from the more solid blue cheeses, such as Stilton, Gorgonzola, and Roquefort.

what to eat

The UK's Department of Health says that the following cheeses are safe to eat: hard cheeses, e.g. Cheddar, Parmesan, Cornish Yarg, Red Leicester, etc.; softer cheeses that do not have any mould or rind and are made from pasteurized milk, e.g. cottage cheese, ricotta, and mozzarella; processed cheese and cheese spreads.

Sometimes it is not easy to tell the type of cheese, so it is best to check the label. If you are not sure, play safe and don't eat it.

milk & cream

It is best to avoid raw milk from the time that you start planning to have a baby...

what to avoid

The UK's Department of Health advises avoiding all "raw" milk and cream from cows, sheep, or goats. Raw milk has not been pasteurized and may contain bacteria and other organisms which can cause illness. In particular, unpasteurized goat's and sheep's milk may contain the parasite *Toxoplasma gondii*.

Raw cow's milk carries the following warning: "This milk has not been heat-treated and may therefore contain organisms harmful to health." This warning has now been extended to include raw sheep's and goat's milk.

It is best to avoid raw milk from the time that you start planning to have baby to the time that you finish breastfeeding.

what to eat

Pasteurized milk and cream are readily available and are perfectly safe, whether they come from cows, sheep, or goats.

eggs

It is advisable to choose organic eggs, since their production requires a more stringently controlled food production system which has a high standard of hygiene.

what to avoid

The salmonella bacteria are most likely to be passed on through contaminated poultry and eggs. This applies to all types of eggs, whether they are duck, quail, goose, etc. Approximately one egg in every 450 in the UK is contaminated with salmonella.

It is advisable to choose organic eggs, since their production requires a more stringently controlled food production system which has a high standard of hygiene.

Avoid eating foods that contain raw or partly cooked egg, for example, mousse, homemade mayonnaise, sorbets, soft meringues, icing, and cheesecakes.

what to eat

The good news is that thorough cooking often eliminates salmonella, so it is fine to eat eggs that have been cooked so thoroughly that the egg yolks are hard. If you need to make a recipe that normally uses raw egg, try replacing the raw egg with pasteurized egg products which are available in supermarkets – pasteurization heats the eggs and kills the bacteria. While homemade mayonnaise should not be eaten, bought mayonnaise is often safe to eat as long as it is made with pasteurized eggs, so check the label.

meat

raw or rare meats: what to avoid

Undercooked and raw poultry and meat may be contaminated with bacteria, which can cause food poisoning. These bacteria are destroyed when you cook food at high temperatures. Raw meat may also contain toxoplasma (*see* page 66), an organism which can, in rare cases, affect an unborn child.

It is also best to avoid foods preserved in nitrates, such as smoked or cured meats, frankfurters, salami, and luncheon meats (*Ref. 3.1*).

what to eat

The UK's Department of Health advises cooking all meat and poultry, including burgers and sausages, until the juices run clear and there is no remaining blood or pinkness. This is because any bacteria that may be present are destroyed when exposed to high temperatures. The UK's Health Development Agency supports this statement.

Wash your hands thoroughly when handling raw meat and store raw foods separately from cooked foods.

liver: what to avoid

There is a risk to pregnant women of excessive intake of vitamin A in the form of retinol from liver and liver products. In recent years, the vitamin A content of animal liver has increased considerably, probably due to changes in feeding practices. A 100-g portion of liver can contain between 20,000–40,000 mcg of vitamin A, depending on the animal.

This is obviously unacceptably high when you consider that the upper safe level is 8,000 to 10,000 mcg per day for pregnant women. The Department of Health therefore recommends that women who are trying to become pregnant or who are pregnant should avoid eating liver and liver products such as pâté and liver sausage.

In addition, meat pâté may contain high levels of listeria.

Undercooked and raw poultry and meat may be contaminated with bacteria, which can cause food poisoning.

seafood & fish

what to avoid

The Department of Health advises pregnant women not to eat oysters. They are also advised to avoid shelled seafood such as prawns, mussels, and crabs, unless they are a part of a hot meal and have been thoroughly cooked. When raw, these foods may be contaminated with harmful bacteria and viruses.

It is also recommended that pregnant women limit their intakes of predatory fish such as swordfish, fresh tuna, and shark – all of which are mercury-rich – to no more than one serving per month. However, levels of mercury in canned tuna are lower, so it is fine to eat a couple of cans per week.

Do not eat fish from contaminated waters or tropical fish such as grouper, amberjack, and mahi-mahi. It is also best to avoid foods preserved in nitrates – for example, smoked fish.

what to eat

Because unwanted chemicals collect in fatty tissue, it is best to eat lean seafood such as sole, flounder, haddock, Pacific halibut, ocean perch, pollack, and cod. Salmon is also fine. Seafood should be well cooked.

Most fresh fish from reputable suppliers and restaurants are safe to eat during pregnancy.

salads

...avoid ready-made dressed salads, such as potato salad and coleslaw...

what to avoid

Pre-prepared and packaged salads – available in bags from supermarkets – may contain listeria bacteria. Also avoid ready-made dressed salads, such as potato salad and coleslaw for the same reasons. In addition, salad leaves that have not been thoroughly washed may carry the toxoplasmosis parasite (*see page 66*).

what to eat

Make your own salads. The British Department of Health recommends that all salad ingredients should be washed well in order to remove any soil or dirt. It is also advisable to wash thoroughly any soil from your hands and kitchen surfaces.

convenience foods

what to avoid

The UK's Health Development Agency advises that raw or undercooked ready-prepared meals should be avoided due to the risk of listeria. This bacteria has been found in cooked-chilled meals and also in ready-to-eat poultry, including plain roast chicken. It is important to note that listeria bacteria can multiply even at low temperatures, such as inside a supermarket chill cabinet or your refrigerator.

what to eat

The UK's Department of Health advises that ready-prepared meals can be eaten, but stresses that they must be reheated until they are piping hot throughout. The Health Development Agency reinforces this stance.

The following guidelines can help you store and cook foods properly.

- Whenever possible, keep chilled convenience foods cool, preferably in an insulated bag or box during travel and transfer them straight to the fridge.
- Keep your fridge temperature between 0° and 4°C.
- Always eat foods by their "best before" date; this way, any bacteria that the foods do contain may not have multiplied to dangerous levels.
- Follow instructions on reheating the foods carefully. Because listeria bacteria are not killed by low temperatures, thorough reheating is essential. If you are using an oven, allow time for it to warm up. If you are using a microwave, check that you are using the cooking times appropriate to the microwave's power level. Always follow instructions about standing times or stirring; this helps to distribute the heat evenly.
- Before eating food, check that the middle is piping hot.

Follow instructions on reheating the foods carefully. Because listeria bacteria are not killed by low temperatures, thorough reheating is essential.

nuts

...exclusive breastfeeding for the first six months helps decrease the risk of allergies in our baby's early years.

what to avoid

The British Department of Health recommends avoiding peanuts if you, your baby's father, or one of your previous children suffers from any allergic conditions. These include eczema, asthma, hay fever, and any allergic response (rashes, itches, and bumps) after eating food such as strawberries, shellfish, or peanuts.

Peanut allergy is a growing problem in the UK. Approximately one in 200 four-year-old children has a peanut allergy; most of these children will develop the problem before their third birthday. In rare cases, peanut allergy can cause a severe reaction called anaphylactic shock, which can be life-threatening.

Before an allergy can develop, a child first has to come into contact with small traces of peanut. This initial contact can cause a future reaction when the child eats peanuts or foods containing peanuts. Some experts now think that this initial sensitization may occur during pregnancy, when a tiny amount of the peanut protein crosses the placenta. There is no definitive evidence to prove this yet, and further research is needed.

However, because peanut allergy is an increasing problem, the government has advised that women with an allergic reaction to peanuts or women who know of a family member that has an allergic reaction to peanuts should avoid them while pregnant or breastfeeding.

Breastfeeding gives your baby protection against many infections; exclusive breastfeeding for the first six months helps decrease the risk of allergies in your baby's early years. However, if you eat peanuts, there is a small chance that your baby will come into contact with traces of peanut through your milk.

As stated above, if you decide to avoid peanuts while pregnant or breastfeeding, you need to avoid not only peanuts themselves – which are also sometimes called monkey nuts or groundnuts – but also any products that may contain them. These include peanut butter, cereals, cakes, muesli, biscuits, some salad dressings, ice cream, and breads.

Always read the packaging label carefully for information on ingredients. Supermarkets should be able to provide a list of the nut-free products it produces and sells.

When ordering dishes in restaurants, either ask if peanuts have been included or choose a simple meal which contains no "hidden" ingredients.

what to eat
For everyone else, nuts and seeds are a great source of protein, fat, B vitamins, and iron. Because they are so high in fat, they also tend to be high in calories, so it is worth bearing this in mind when you eat them as a snack.

...nuts and seeds are a great source of protein, fat, B vitamins, and iron.

foods & comfort

nausea & sickness

Try drinking rice water. Take small sips of the warm water left in the saucepan after you have boiled rice.

what it is

Morning sickness, which tends to affect seven in 10 women, is a feeling of nausea and, in some cases, vomiting, which often occurs in the morning but can happen at any time during the day. It is caused by hormonal and metabolic changes and usually lasts no longer than the first three months. However, some women can spend their whole nine months feeling and being sick. If you go for more than a day without being able to keep anything down, it is a good idea to visit your doctor or dietician.

how to avoid it

Some of the following suggestions may work for you.

● Use fresh root ginger – known to help relieve nausea – in cooking, or drink ginger tea.

● Peppermint, ginger, and camomile herb teas are also very soothing.

● Some fizzy drinks, for example, ginger ale, are also good at relieving nausea.

● Try drinking rice water. Take small sips of the warm water left in the saucepan after you have boiled rice.

● Try to eat something, such as crackers, plain toast, dry cereal, or anything else that may appeal before getting out of bed in the morning. This will help keep blood-sugar levels steady. Resist chocolate, buttery, or creamy biscuits, since these often aggravate nausea.

• An empty stomach can make nausea worse, so don't go for long periods without eating; eat frequent small meals or snacks. Fruit and seeds make great snacks. See pages 126–31 for more snack ideas.

• Try to avoid high-fat and fried foods, which are particularly difficult to digest. Starchy foods such as bread, pasta, rice, and potatoes are far gentler on the system.

• Make sure your diet is as varied and balanced as possible. One school of thought maintains that morning sickness only occurs in women whose nutrition is less than optimum (Ref. 3.2).

• One possible explanation for morning sickness is that the body is trying to get rid of toxins.

• Women low in B_6 and zinc may have a higher risk of suffering from morning sickness (Ref. 3.3). See page 55 for foods containing vitamin B_6.

• Avoid all sugar, refined foods, and high-fat junk food which contain large quantities of additives and preservatives.

• Drink lots of water between meals.

• Decrease consumption of coffee and tea. They can aggravate nausea and vomiting.

• Avoid alcohol and cigarettes.

• Avoid strong smells.

• Try to get some fresh air prior to eating. If you have the time, a quick stroll before food is a good idea.

supplements

According to Dr Pfeiffer and Nim Barnes of the Foresight Association (see page 9), "The nauseated woman is usually deficient in both zinc and B_6. Both are needed for growing tissues of any kind, and the foetus and uterus make extraordinary demands on the mother's supply. We have had many pregnant patients who had difficulties with previous pregnancies go through a pregnancy on a zinc and B_6 regime with no difficulties."

If nausea and sickness persist it may be worthwhile getting your GP to check your nutritional status to assess if further supplementation is necessary.

One possible explanation for morning sickness is that the body is trying to get rid of toxins.

weight

It is advised that you lose excess weight well in advance of your planned pregnancy...

It is possible that your pre-pregnancy weight can have a direct impact on the birth weight of your baby.

Body Mass Index, or BMI, is an index of a person's weight in relation to height. It is calculated by dividing your weight (in kilograms) by the square of your height (in metres): $BMI = kg/m^2$

Weight in pounds (one stone = 14 lb) can be converted to kilograms by multiplying pounds by 0.4536. Height in inches can be converted to metres by multiplying inches by 0.0254. A BMI of 23 to 24 is considered good for general health, fertility, and birth weight (*Ref. 3.5*).

underweight

If you have a low BMI, this may also be an indication of a poor nutritional status, which is linked to low birth weight. A study of underweight women and pregnancy outcome showed that underweight women (BMI below 19.1 kg/m^2) had a three-fold increased risk of having a low-birth-weight baby.

overweight

Women who are overweight when they conceive (BMIs over 30) are more likely to face pregnancy problems such as hypertension, pre-eclampsia, and gestational diabetes. It is therefore advised to lose excess weight well in advance of your planned pregnancy, allowing at least two or three months of good, well-balanced nutrition before conception. It is not advised to attempt to diet when pregnant.

normal Body Mass Index (BMI) gradations

	BMI
Underweight	less than 20
Acceptable weight	20–24.9
Overweight	25–29.9
Fat	30–39.9
Very fat	greater than 40

Women who are overweight may find that they only gain a small amount as their bodies intuitively know that they do not need extra fat storage.

weight gain

How much you gain during your pregnancy depends on your height and how much you weighed before you conceived. If you were underweight, you are likely to gain between 13 kg and 18 kg; if you were an average pre-pregnancy weight, you should gain between 11 kg and 16 kg; and if you were overweight, between 7 kg and 11 kg. If you are having twins, the average weight gain is about 16 kg to 20 kg. (*Ref. 3.6*).

The increased blood volume, breast and uterine tissue, amniotic fluid, baby, placenta, and fluid retention – all products of pregnancy – account for about 4.5 kg to 7 kg of normal pregnancy weight gain. Women who are overweight may find that they only gain a small amount as their bodies intuitively know that they do not need extra fat storage (*Ref. 3.7*).

If you are concerned that you are not gaining enough weight, try the following suggestions.
• Eat small meals often.
• Try to ensure that the meals are as full of energy as possible. Make sure that your diet consists of a variety of protein, carbohydrates, and good fats.

• Also eat nutrient-rich foods such as cheese, milk, full-fat yoghurt, fish, cream, meat, and butter. Dried fruits, e.g. apricots, figs, and prunes, are good snack foods.

If you are concerned that you are gaining too much weight too soon, reduce the number of calories you eat and concentrate on eating nutrient-rich foods.
• When cooking, use a minimum amount of fat.
• Snack on fresh, poached, or dried fruit, either on its own or with some fromage frais or yoghurt.
• *See* the government's guide to healthy eating (page 35).

indigestion

what it is

Heartburn is very common in the later stages of pregnancy. This can be caused partly by the baby's body pressing on your stomach. Also, the hormone changes during pregnancy can cause the muscles at the top of your stomach to over-relax, making it more likely that its acidic contents will leak into your oesophagus. The presence of these acidic juices in your oesophagus causes an acidic, unpleasant sensation – heartburn. This complaint is often made worse at night, when you are lying down.

how to avoid it

• It is important not to rely on medication, which can interfere with absorption of vitamins and minerals.
• Avoid large meals. Choose small, frequent meals or snacks instead.
• Avoid eating fatty foods on an empty stomach. Also avoid foods that you find hard to digest.
• Take time when eating, and chew food properly.
• Sit up straight when eating and avoid activity just after a meal.
• Fizzy drinks, citrus fruits, soda, caffeine, alcohol, processed meats, and spicy, highly seasoned, fried, and fatty foods can make the problem worse.
• Avoid drinking too much when you are eating.
• Try to gain a sensible amount of weight (see page 79).
• Do not eat too late at night.
• Sleep with your head propped up a little.
• Sip settling drinks such as peppermint or ginger tea, or ice water.
• Some experts advise avoiding antacid preparations, unless recommended by your doctor, midwife, or chemist. Some of these contain high levels of aluminium or sodium, which are not ideal for pregnant women.

It is important not to rely on medication, which can interfere with absorption of vitamins and minerals.

cravings

what they are

Cravings usually occur in the first and last three months of pregnancy, when the body experiences dramatic changes. Some women experience cravings for the strangest foods, about 85 percent of women report at least one food craving during pregnancy. American Babycenter.com users confessed to wanting pickles wrapped in cheese, salsa spooned straight out of the jar, and even steak fat (*Ref. 3.10*). "Quite a lot of cravings are for out-of-season foods and foods which bear no resemblance to things previously liked by women," says Cornian Casey-Hardman, a senior midwife at The Liverpool Women's Hospital (*Ref. 3.11*). Usually such cravings are not a problem, as long as you are still able to eat a well-balanced diet. You may also experience strong aversions to fatty foods, alcohol, tea, and coffee.

Cravings can be interpreted in several ways. Later on in pregnancy, some women develop cravings for hot, spicy food. This can be because their senses of taste has reduced, so they crave more highly flavoured foods.

...about 85 percent of women report at least one food craving...

There is also some evidence that particularly strange cravings for substances such as coal are due to a lack of certain key nutrients in the system, while others may be due to comfort eating.

A possible explanation for cravings is a change in taste and smell during pregnancy. Cravings may be caused by an impaired sense of taste, while aversions are more likely to be due to an altered sense of smell.

Some cravings and aversions can arise subconsciously if you are trying to improve your diet and avoid unhealthy food and drink.

There is also research that indicates that hormonal changes can cause cravings. This has also been shown in non-food cravings such as smells or an increased desire for sex.

constipation & piles

what they are

Constipation can occur when extra hormones produced in pregnancy cause the intestine to relax and become less efficient. Coupled with pressure from the baby, this can, over time, lead to the development of haemorrhoids or piles (varicose veins of the anus). Sometimes piles only appear for the first time during labour as you strain to push your baby out. Luckily, pregnancy piles nearly always disappear within three months of giving birth.

Another reason that pregnancy also makes women more prone to haemorrhoids – and, similarly, to bleeding gums – is because the amount of blood circulating through your body increases. This causes all your veins to become dilated. In particular, the veins below the level of your uterus are susceptible to becoming varicose – abnormally swollen or dilated – as the uterus places increased pressure upon them.

how to avoid them

● Eat plenty of fresh fruit, vegetables,and wholegrain cereals.
● Eat dried fruit.
● Drink lots of water – at least two litres a day.
● Swimming and other light exercise can also help.

Sometimes piles only appear for the first time during labour ... pregnancy piles nearly always disappear within three months of giving birth.

anaemia

what it is

A mild form of anaemia may be present in one in three pregnant women. Symptoms include pallor, tiredness, a sore tongue, unusual tiredness, and feeling as if the weight of the world is on your shoulders (*Ref. 3.12*).

how to avoid it

Anaemia is usually the result of a low level of iron, although vitamin B_{12}, folic acid, manganese, and vitamin B_6 deficiency can also contribute (*see* the section on iron, page 51).

insomnia

what it is

Not being able to sleep at night is something that almost all pregnant women experience at some point during the last few weeks of their pregnancies. This is hardly surprising – the size of your tummy makes it difficult to get comfortable, You may be getting up several times to go to the toilet, your baby may be kicking, or you may be woken by cramp. You may also be kept awake by worry, or be woken by disturbing dreams.

Pregnant women barely sleep enough for one person, let alone two, according to the US National Sleep Foundation (NSF) 1998 Women and Sleep Poll (WSP). A whopping 79 percent of women who took part in the poll said their sleep is more disturbed during pregnancy than at other times.

The study states that many pregnant women make up for their sleep deficits by napping – they are almost twice as likely to be sleepy during the day than other women. Half of pregnant or recently pregnant women – 51 percent – take at least one weekday nap, and 60 percent take at least one nap at weekends.

how to avoid it

- Lie on your side with a pillow under your bump and another between your knees.
- Practice relaxation exercises, particularly breathing slowly and deeply when trying to get to sleep,
- Have a warm bath before going to bed.
- Have a warm, milky drink before going to bed.
- Have a massage at bedtime.
- Do some gentle exercise – for example, walking or swimming – during the day.
- Just as with any significant problems in sleeping, rest as much as possible during the day to make up for the sleep lost at night.

Have a warm, milky drink before going to bed.

cramps

what they are

Cramps are very likely to be caused by an imbalance of calcium and magnesium. Other possible causes of pregnancy-related leg cramps include the following:

- an excess of phosphorus and a shortage of calcium circulating in the blood;
- the pressure of the expanding uterus on the nerves leading to the legs;
- decreased circulation in the legs from the pressure of the baby on blood vessels;
- tired muscles. The extra weight on your leg muscles can lead to night cramps, which can wake you out of a sound sleep. Leg cramps normally occur between three and nine months of pregnancy (*Ref. 3.13*).

Other possible causes of pregnancy-related leg cramps include... an excess of phosphorus and a shortage of calcium circulating in the blood.

how to avoid them

If you find yourself with cramp, try the following steps to relieve the pain.
- Walk. This may be uncomfortable at first, but it helps relieve cramping.
- Stand with your legs straight and bend the toes toward your head, without bending your knees.
- Try resting with your legs raised on pillows or the arm of a sofa.
- Avoid massaging your legs if they have red or especially painful spots.
- Stretching your calf muscles several times before going to bed can help.
- Avoid standing for long periods or sitting with crossed legs.
- Eat calcium-rich foods.
- Avoid soft drinks – they contain a lot of phosphorus.
- Moderate exercise may help.
- Avoid wearing constrictive clothing of any type.
- Wear shoes with low heels.
- Rest, especially if standing for long hours during the day.

drugs & safety

hot drinks

caffeine

Research is inconsistent about the effects of drinking more than five cups of coffee a day, which is why experts don't always agree on how to advise pregnant women. My advice would be to drink up to one or two cups of coffee or equivalent a day, and if possible, to cut it out completely. Decaffeinated drinks are not recommended as they can contain other stimulants and possibly harmful residues, such as pesticides (*Ref. 3.14*).

A mug of instant coffee contains 100 mg of caffeine, a mug of ground coffee up to 150 mg, and a mug of tea between 80 and 100 mg. The substance is also present in cola-based drinks, chocolate, and cocoa.

The effects of caffeine during pregnancy are not fully known. Although many experts believe that ingesting too much caffeine may contribute to the risk of low-birth-weight babies.

The *Journal of the American Medical Association* reported a study which found that the risk of miscarriage doubled in women who drank two or three cups of ground coffee or its equivalent daily (*Ref. 3.15*).

Other studies have linked miscarriage, low birth weight and birth defects to large amounts of caffeine. However, much of this research failed to take into account other risk factors such as smoking and alcohol intake, which can also lead to complications in pregnancy, labour, and delivery.

Caffeine is a stimulant; it increases your heart rate and metabolism, which in turn affects your developing baby. But while constant stress is not healthy, brief bouts of foetal stress, such as that your baby would feel after you've drunk a cup of coffee, won't cause him or her any harm – it briefly boosts your heart rate and metabolism.

Caffeine is also a diuretic, and it can interfere with the absorption of certain nutrients.

what to avoid

Coffee, tea, colas, and chocolate in large quantities. Some over-the-counter drugs including headache and cold tablets, stay-awake medications, and allergy remedies may also contain caffeine. If you are consuming a lot of caffeine daily, it is best to wean yourself off the substance gradually.

herbal teas

Look on packaging labels for contents that may normally be part of your diet, such as mint or orange extracts. Choose them over unfamiliar substances such as black cohosh root or mugwort.

alcohol

Experts are not able to say how much or how little alcohol can harm a developing baby. Danger levels are most likely different for each individual woman because everyone metabolizes alcohol differently. It is felt that the effects of alcohol are greater in women who smoke, consume large amounts of caffeine, and have a poor diet.

Some health bodies, including the Royal College of Physicians, recommend that pregnant women play it safe by steering clear of alcohol completely. Others, such as the Royal College of Obstetricians and Gynaecologists, recommend that women should simply limit their intake to one unit of alcohol per day (half a pint of beer or cider, a glass of wine, a small glass of sherry, or a single measure of spirits).

The British Department of Health advises that to minimize risk to unborn children, pregnant women should drink no more than one or two units of alcohol once or twice a week, and should avoid heavy drinking sessions.

Foresight (see page 9) takes the view that both partners should abstain from alcohol in the preconception phase, and that women should continue to stay away from alcohol throughout pregnancy (*see* page 29 for more information on fertility and alcohol).

Professor Matthew Kaufman, an expert on early embryology, says of alcohol: "The only thing we can say is [that] 'safe' is none at all until child-bearing is over." This is supported by the Surgeon General of the United States: "Pregnant women and those planning a pregnancy should abstain from the use of alcohol."

The World Health Organization, agrees: "No alcohol during pregnancy is the only safe limit."

what to do and why

Toxins from alcohol are at their most dangerous during the first few weeks of pregnancy, so it is a good idea to stop drinking alcohol at least two weeks before conception.

It is thought that alcohol crosses the placenta freely and babies receive the alcohol before it is broken down by the mother's liver. A baby's own liver only starts forming some four weeks after conception and cannot deal with the alcohol, so damage may occur (*Ref. 3.16*).

Alcohol is sometimes described as an "anti-nutrient" because its consumption can lead to malabsorption, or increased urinary excretion of nutrients needed during pregnancy – in particular, thiamine, zinc, vitamin A, and folic acid.

However, if you have discovered that you are pregnant and you have been drinking, try not to worry. A great many women have had a drink or two before they knew they were pregnant and their babies have been fine.

proven risks

Women who drink over six units of alcohol per day are at risk of having babies with foetal alcohol syndrome (FAS). Children born with FAS may suffer from mental and growth retardation, behavioural problems, and facial and heart defects.

Babies of women who drink more than two glasses of alcohol a day throughout their pregnancy are more likely to have problems with learning speech, attention span, language, and hyperactivity than babies of women who did not drink. These are known as Foetal Alcohol Effects (FAE).

nicotine

what to do and why

Many professional experts advise stopping smoking long before you try to conceive. If it is not possible to stop completely, it is advised that you cut down. This applies to both the mother- and father-to-be.

In the US, smoking during pregnancy has been identified as the single most important preventable determinant of low birth weight and perinatal death. As well as infertility (see page 30), other links that have been formed between smoking and pregnancy outcome include miscarriage, premature delivery, physical abnormalities at birth, and stillbirth (Ref. 3.17).

smoking and miscarriage

Expectant mothers who smoke may have lower levels of hormones, which has led researchers to believe that this could be one reason why smoking results in ill effects to unborn babies. Miscarriages are known to be influenced by hormonal changes.

smoking and birth weight

The higher the number of cigarettes smoked by the expectant mother, the lower the birth weight is likely to be. This effect on birth size is caused by the cigarette's ability to slow down the rate of growth of the foetus. It may do this by damaging the DNA. In turn, this has consequences for mental and physical development.

fathers and smoking

A large study in Germany has shown that even when only the father smokes, there is an increased incidence of pregnancy and birth problems (Ref. 3.19).

Although research has shown that multivitamin supplementation appears to offer some protection against the risk of low birth weight, it is strongly advisable simply to stop smoking altogether.

how to quit

The good news is that more people succeed in stopping smoking when planning to become pregnant or during pregnancy than at other times – women wish to stop because they want to give their babies the best possible chance while in their womb.

Your local Citizens Advice Bureau should be able to provide you with the names and addresses of local groups that can help you to quit. See "Useful Addresses", page 143, for details of Action on Smoking and Health.

pregnancy recipes

three meals
a day

...if you eat small meals frequently, you are more likely to feel good, keep your energy levels constant and eat a greater variety of nutrients throughout the day...

I have developed recipes for breakfasts, lunches, suppers, and snacks that rely heavily on fresh fruit, vegetables, and seeds. These recipe ideas are based around fresh fruits, vegetables and stamina foods such as wholegrains, pulses (beans, lentils etc) fish and meat – all of which provide a variety of nutrients needed for a healthy pregnancy.

Breakfast is too important to miss. Studies show that if you eat a high-carbohydrate breakfast, it can result in a lower overall intake of fat throughout the day. By skipping breakfast, you are more likely to binge on high-fat foods later.

Eat a good lunch that will not leave you feeling too full or heavy. Lunches high in carbohydrates are difficult for the system to digest and can put strain on the body, leaving you feeling tired. The lunches in this book are all relatively light, providing a good mix of protein, carbohydrates and lots of vitamins and minerals.

Aim to eat supper a good few hours before going to bed so that your bodies have time to digest the food before you sleep.

I believe that if you eat small meals frequently you are more likely to feel good, keep your energy levels constant and eat a greater variety of nutrients throughout the day. For this reason, I have developed a few snack recipes for you to try.

When it comes to choosing ingredients, go for fresh and, wherever possible, seasonal and organic. For information about organic foods, *see* pages 38-39.

breakfasts

smoothies

 ### strawberry shake

Serves: 2

200 g strawberries

1 banana, peeled and chopped

fortified soya drink (milk alternative), enough to make a good consistency

a little unrefined sugar, to taste (optional)

Strawberries are a good source of **betacarotene**, which helps to boost the immune system. Bananas are a good source of **folic acid** and fortified soya drink provides **protein**.

1 Throw the fruit into a food processor or blender with a little soya drink and whiz until smooth.

2 Add enough milk to make a smooth, thick (but not too thick) shake. Add sugar to taste.

 ### mango & melon smoothie

Serves: 2

1 mango

½ melon, e.g. ogen or cantaloupe, peeled and deseeded

sparkling water (optional)

A whole mango provides more than the daily requirement of **vitamin C**. Melons provide **folic acid**, which helps to prevent birth defects.

1 Cut the mango either side of the stone, peel the flesh, and put into a food processor or blender.
2 Add the melon flesh and whiz until smooth. Add sparkling water if you want to dilute it slightly.

fibre-boost fruit smoothies

Serves: 2

250 ml semi-skimmed milk or fortified soya drink

4 tbsp natural yoghurt

2 tsp runny honey

1 tbsp oat germ

1 tbsp wheat germ

fruit of your choice, e.g. 1 banana, peeled and chopped

or 1 banana, peeled and chopped, handful of raspberries, and handful of blueberries

or 1 banana, peeled and chopped, and 1 passion-fruit, halved and flesh scooped out

or ½ mango, stoned and peeled, and 1 passion-fruit, halved and flesh scooped out

or 6 dried apricots, chopped

Oat germ, wheat germ, and fruit are all great sources of soluble **fibre**, while the milk and yoghurt provide **calcium** and **protein**. The fruit also gives your body a few **vitamins** and **minerals**.

1 Put the first five ingredients with one of the fruit combinations (*see left*) of your choice into a food processor or blender

2 Process until smooth.

papaya, melon, & grape smoothie

Serves: 2–3 (halve the ingredients if you want to make one large drink)

2 papayas
½ cantaloupe
juice of ½ lime
small bunch of seedless grapes
sparkling water

Papapya and cantaloupe are excellent sources of **betacarotene**, which is essential for reproduction and growth. The bubbles in sparkling water can help to alleviate morning sickness.

1 Cut the papayas in half and scoop out the seeds. Peel and put the flesh into a food processor or blender. Scoop the seeds from the melon, peel, and add the melon flesh to the processor or blender.
2 Add the lime juice and grapes, and whiz until smooth. You may need to add sparkling water to make the right consistency.

mango & banana smoothie

Serves: 2

½ mango
½ banana, peeled and chopped
juice of ½ lime
pinch of ground cardamom
250 ml natural yoghurt
100 ml water
a little unrefined brown sugar or honey, to taste
ice cubes (optional)

The banana will supply a good source of energy, and the mango and lime will give you a burst of **vitamin C**, which will help to boost the immune system. Adding yoghurt to a smoothie is a quick and easy way of incorporating **calcium** into the diet.

1 Slice the mango either side of the stone, peel one half, and put the flesh into a food processor or blender. Add the banana, lime juice, cardamom, yoghurt, and water, and whiz for about 30 seconds, until smooth.
2 Pour it into glasses and add sugar or honey to taste and ice cubes, if using.

citrus drink

(diluted with water)

Serves: 2

2 oranges
1 grapefruit
lime juice, to taste
ice cubes (optional)

Wake up with one of these. Oranges, grapefruit, and limes are an excellent source of **vitamin C**, while grapefruit contains pectin, which helps to lower cholesterol levels in the blood.

1 Cut the oranges and grapefruit in half and squeeze out all the juice.
2 Add lime juice to taste and ice cubes, if using. Drink and enjoy.

fruits

mango & strawberries with toasted oats

Serves: 2

40 g organic oats
1 large ripe mango, peeled,
stoned, and chopped
6 strawberries, sliced
juice of ½ lime
100 g Greek yoghurt
honey, to taste

This is an easy way to incorporate more fresh fruit into your diet. Toasting the oats gives them a wonderful crunch and they will help to keep your energy levels up during the morning.

1 Lightly toast the oats in a dry frying pan until lightly golden. Toss the fruit with the lime juice and put into two dishes.

2 Top with yoghurt and the toasted oats. Drizzle with honey.

vanilla roasted fruits

Serves: 4

900 g plums
3 peaches or nectarines
1 vanilla pod
1–2 tbsp golden caster sugar, to taste

These fruits make a great change to fresh fruit, mixed with yoghurt and cereal for breakfast. Alternatively, use to make into a crumble for supper. If the fruit is naturally sweet, add only a little sugar. Choose any fruit in season: plums, nectarines, figs, cherries, pears, and apples all work really well.

1 Preheat the oven to 200°C/ 400°F/gas mark 6. Cut the plums and peaches or nectarines in half, remove the stones, and put the fruit into an ovenproof dish.
2 Cut a slit in the vanilla pod and scrape half the seeds into a bowl; add the sugar, and mix together. Scatter the vanilla sugar over the fruit and roast for approximately 10 minutes, until the fruit is slightly soft, but still holding its shape. Alternatively, put the fruit under a hot grill for five minutes.
3 Serve with yoghurt and cereal, or use as the base for a crumble.

dried fruit compote

Serves: 4

200 ml apple juice

200 ml orange juice

350 g mixed dried fruit, e.g. pears, peaches, prunes, apricots, and figs

handful of raisins

½ tsp ground cinnamon and 1 cinnamon stick

Cooking the dried fruit in juice makes it really plump and sweet. Choose fruit that you like – I used pears, peaches, figs, etc. Alternatively, you could use a bag of mixed dried fruit. This will keep for a few days; cover and store in the fridge.

Mixed dried fruit is a good source of **iron** and **folic acid**. Apple and orange juice are both good sources of **vitamin C**, which improves iron absorption in the body.

1 Put all the ingredients into a pan and bring to the boil.

2 Remove from the heat and leave to cool.

fresh fruit salad with raspberry sauce

Serves: 2

a selection of fresh fruit of your choice, e.g. 1 each mango or nectarine and papaya, prepared and cut into chunks

for the raspberry sauce:

150 g frozen or fresh raspberries or mixed berries

1–2 tsp golden caster sugar

squeeze of lime or lemon juice

yoghurt and sunflower seeds, to serve

Fresh fruit is a good source of **fibre** and **vitamin C**, which helps the body with digestion and absorption of iron. Yoghurt provides **calcium**, which helps with the formation of bones.

Another delicious winning combination is a mixture of melon, papaya, and fresh basil or mint, with a little maple syrup drizzled over the top.

1 Make the sauce; put all the ingredients in a heavy-based saucepan and simmer until the raspberries have turned to a pulp. Taste for sweetness; leave to cool.

2 Scatter your chosen fresh fruit over two plates and drizzle the raspberry sauce over the top, finishing with a dollop of yoghurt and a sprinkling of sunflower seeds.

cereals

nutty fruity bar

Makes: 15

50 g butter

25 g golden caster sugar

75 g golden syrup

250 g jumbo rolled oats

25 g pumpkin seeds, toasted

50 g Brazil nuts, chopped and toasted

40 g dried apricots, roughly chopped

40 g dried mango, cut into small pieces

1 tbsp sesame seeds, toasted

Once you have made these, you can just grab one as and when you choose. They will keep in an airtight container or in the freezer.

These bars are packed with goodness; the oats provide **folic acid**, and the seeds and nuts are good sources of **zinc**, **calcium**, and **iron**.

1 Grease a 20-cm square tin. Preheat the oven to 180°C/350°F/ gas mark 4. Put the butter, sugar, and syrup into a pan and heat until the butter is melted.
2 Add all the other ingredients and mix well. Tip into the greased tin and bake in the oven for 25–30 minutes.

3 Mark into squares and leave to cool in the tin. Cut and store in an airtight container.

creamy porridge

Serves: 4

375 ml milk

375 ml water

75 g organic porridge oats

topping suggestions:

a selection of fresh fruit, chopped into pieces

a couple of spoons of Dried Fruit Compote (page 95) or Vanilla Roasted Fruits (page 94)

chopped banana and dates with a little treacle

a sprinkling of wheat germ and a chopped kiwi fruit with a drizzle of honey

dark muscovado sugar or golden sugar

I find porridge one of the best ways to start the day. The oats provide slow-release energy and **B-complex vitamins**, keeping your energy levels constant through the morning. Always add some soya drink or milk for **protein** and pile fresh or dried fruit on top – whatever is to hand. Traditionally, a little pinch of salt is added, but I prefer it without.

1 Put the milk and water into a saucepan and add the oats. Bring to the boil, reduce to a simmer, and cook for five minutes.
2 Serve the porridge with any one of the suggested toppings.

dried fruit & nut muesli

Makes: 6–8

40 g sunflower seeds

50 g almonds, roughly chopped

75 g whole hazelnuts or cashew nuts, roughly chopped

50 g coconut chips (available from supermarkets) or desiccated coconut

300 g rolled oats

4 tbsp wheat germ

125 g each dried apricots, chopped, and raisins

75 g dried cranberries or blueberries

pinch of freshly grated or ground nutmeg

½ tsp cinnamon

choose milk; soya drink; natural or soya yoghurt; fruit juice and fresh fruit, to serve

This is easy and quick to make, and will last for a good few breakfasts; just keep it in an airtight jar. To make the muesli toddler- or baby-friendly, whiz in a food processor to a powder. However, avoid giving it to babies or toddlers with nut allergies.

Oats, wheat germ, and dried fruit are all rich in **fibre**, which helps with **digestion**, and nuts and seeds are a good source of **protein**. Dried cranberries help to fight bladder, kidney, and urinary-tract infections.

1 Dry-fry the seeds and nuts in a frying pan over a medium heat, stirring constantly, until they begin to brown – this only takes a couple of minutes. Transfer to a bowl.

2 Dry-fry the coconut chips or desiccated coconut for a minute until lightly golden. Add to the bowl of seeds and nuts. Add all the other ingredients to the bowl and mix everything together.

3 Serve with your choice of milk, yoghurt, or fruit juice and fresh fruit.

cooked breakfasts

kippers with wholemeal toast

Serves: 2

2 fresh, plump kipper fillets
knob of butter
handful of flat-leaf parsley, roughly chopped
freshly ground black pepper

Granary toast, to serve

If you have never cooked kippers before, it is worth remembering that grilling the fish will intensify its flavour and give it a slight crust. Poaching, on the other hand, tends to lessen its flavour but will make it more succulent. Kippers are a very good source of **essential fats**, which are important for a developing foetus.

1 Bring a large pan of water to the boil. Add the kippers, return to the boil and remove from the heat. Leave for three minutes, drain well.

2 Dot with a little butter and sprinkle with parsley and freshly ground black pepper. Serve immediately with toast.

passion-fruit & pineapple muffins

Makes: 12

100 g butter
90 g soft brown sugar
125 ml vanilla yoghurt
2 eggs
8 passion-fruit, halved
432 g can crushed pineapple
zest of ½ lime
juice of 1 lime
525 g self-raising flour

Anything can be thrown into muffins. But these work particularly well because the pineapple helps to keep them wonderfully moist.

1 Preheat the oven to 180°C/350°F/gas mark 4. Grease the muffin tins.
2 Whiz the butter, sugar, yoghurt, and eggs in a food processor until smooth. Add the passion-fruit pulp, pineapple, and lime zest and juice.
3 Fold in the flour, spoon into the muffin tins, and bake for 25–30 minutes.

sweet potato frittata

Serves: 2

150 g sweet potato, peeled and chopped into small pieces

50 g spinach

75 g peas

2 tbsp olive oil

½ onion, peeled and finely chopped

4 eggs

freshly ground black pepper

Sweet potatoes are a very good source of **betacarotene**, which helps to boost the immune system. Spinach is a very good source of **iron** and **folic acid**, and eggs provide **protein**.

1 Bring a pan of water to the boil, add the sweet potato, and cook for about 10–15 minutes, until tender. Drain and whiz in a food processor or blender until puréed.

2 Heat a little water in a pan and add the spinach and peas. Cook for one to two minutes, until the spinach has wilted, then drain.

3 Heat half the oil in a small frying pan and sauté the onion until soft.

4 In a bowl, whisk the eggs, add the onion, puréed sweet potato, spinach, and peas, and give it a quick stir without totally blending everything together. Season with a little freshly ground black pepper.

5 Heat the rest of the oil in a small frying pan, turn the heat down, and pour the egg mixture into the pan. Leave to cook until the egg is almost set (about five minutes). Preheat a grill to high and finish cooking the frittata under the grill. Serve in wedges.

lunches

wraps

cream cheese & spinach

Serves: 2

2 flour tortillas

cream cheese

sunblush tomatoes (available from Sainsbury's deli counter) or cherry tomatoes, halved

2 handfuls of baby spinach leaves, washed and dried

freshly ground black pepper

Tortillas are a source of **fibre**, which helps with digestion. Cream cheese provides **calcium**, which helps strengthen bones. Spinach leaves are a good source of **folic acid**, which helps prevent birth defects in early pregnancy.

1 Spread the flour tortillas with cream cheese. Cover with sunblush tomatoes or cherry tomato halves and spinach leaves, and wrap up.

2 If you fancy them warm, wrap in foil and put into a hot oven for five to 10 minutes. Otherwise, eat them as they are.

herby cannellini

Serves: 2–3

175 g canned cannellini beans, drained and rinsed

125 g can mackerel or tuna, drained

½ tsp finely chopped rosemary

a few basil leaves, shredded

1 each small celery stick, tomato, and shallot, peeled; all finely chopped

handful of baby gem lettuce leaves, finely shredded

2–3 flour tortillas

for the dressing:

2 tbsp red-wine vinegar

3 tbsp extra-virgin olive oil

1 clove garlic, peeled and finely chopped

sea salt and freshly ground black pepper

This would also be delicious served with warm new potatoes and a rocket and watercress salad. Another good bean idea is to mix together canned red kidney beans, cream cheese, sliced spring onions, and freshly chopped coriander.

Cannellini beans are an excellent source of **protein** and **fibre**, which provide energy and help with digestion. Canned fish is excellent for **calcium**, helping the body with growth and development.

1 Bring a pan of water to the boil, add the beans, and blanch for a few minutes. Drain and transfer to a bowl. Mash the beans slightly.
2 Mix together the dressing ingredients and add to the beans in the bowl with all the remaining ingredients, except the lettuce and tortillas. Mix thoroughly and season to taste.
3 Scatter the lettuce leaves over the tortillas, cover with the bean spread, and roll up the wraps. Cut in half and serve.

mozzarella, caramelized red onion, & rocket

Serves: 3–4

2 tbsp olive oil
3 red onions, peeled and finely sliced
1 tbsp soft brown sugar
2-3 tsp balsamic vinegar
50 g wild rocket
5 flour tortillas
200 g mozzarella, thinly sliced

Be creative with other fillings; tortillas are great with lots of different flavours. Try meats, cheeses, pestos, and roasted tomatoes. There is a fine line between too much filling and not quite enough – if you are too generous, the wraps don't stay neatly rolled, but skimp and you feel slightly cheated.

Mozzarella is a very good source of **calcium**, which helps to keep bones strong. Wild rocket provides **iron** and **folic acid**, which aid in growth and development.

1 Heat the oil in a frying pan, add the onions, and cook gently for 15 minutes, until starting to caramelize. Add the sugar and balsamic vinegar. Cook for another 10 minutes, until the onions are sweet and sticky.

2 Lay the rocket on the tortillas, arrange a few slices of mozzarella strips in the middle of the tortillas, and cover with a layer of caramelized onions.

3 Roll up the tortillas and wrap in cling film. Refrigerate for at least 30 minutes before serving. Cut each wrap in half and serve.

sandwiches

pesto tuna with tomato & watercress

Serves: 2

200 g tuna canned in oil, drained

2–3 tbsp fresh pesto – to taste, depending on the pesto used

squeeze of lemon juice

freshly ground black pepper

2 chunks of baguette or rolls

2 ripe tomatoes, sliced

handful of watercress leaves

This recipe makes two sandwiches – halve the quantity if you only want one.

Tuna provides **phosphorus**, while baguettes offer **complex carbohydrates** – both help to produce energy. Tomatoes are an excellent source of **vitamin C**, which helps the healing processes in the body.

1 Put the tuna into a bowl, add the pesto, lemon juice, and pepper to taste, and mix together.
2 Spread this mixture onto the chunks of baguette or into the rolls. Cover with the tomato slices and watercress, and the other slices of bread. Wrap up and take to work.

parmesan, pear, & rocket with a balsamic dressing

Serves: 1–2

1 ripe pear

2 granary rolls or bread of your choice

handful each of rocket and watercress

handful of Parmesan cheese shavings

for the dressing:

1 tbsp balsamic vinegar

2 tbsp extra-virgin olive oil

a little squeeze of lime juice

freshly ground black pepper

Pear and bread are both sources of **fibre**, which help with the digestive system. Rocket and watercress both provide **vitamin C**, which helps to boost the immune system.

1 Core the pear, cut into slices, and put into the rolls or onto the bread. Add the rocket, watercress, and Parmesan.
2 Mix together the dressing ingredients and drizzle as much or as little as you fancy into the rolls or onto the bread.

smoked mackerel with horseradish & apple

Serves: 2–3

2–3 smoked mackerel fillets, skinned

2–3 tbsp creamed horseradish

slices of rye or Granary bread

2 apples, cored and sliced

juice of 1 lime

freshly ground black pepper

Oily fish are great sources of **essential fatty acids**, which help with the growth process. Apples and limes are good sources of **vitamin C**, which boosts the immune system.

1 Flake the fish into large pieces, spread the horseradish onto slices of rye or granary bread. Top with the mackerel fillets.

2 Toss the apple slices in a bowl with the lime juice, arrange on top of the fish and season with pepper.

fennel & pepper

Serves: 2

1 fennel bulb

4 slices sun-dried tomato loaf

2 tbsp black olive or sun-dried tomato purée

3 red peppers, raw or roasted, deseeded and thinly sliced

for the dressing:

1 tsp Dijon mustard

juice of ½ lemon

2 tbsp extra-virgin olive oil

handful of fresh flat-leaf parsley, finely chopped

sea salt and freshly ground black pepper

Whenever possible, try to pack raw vegetables into your sandwiches. Raw fennel is crisp, juicy, and has a liquorice flavour; you will need to keep it very thinly sliced to make sure that the flavour is not too strong.

The sun-dried tomato loaf contains **fibre**, which helps with digestion. Red peppers are a very good source of **vitamin C**, which helps boost the body's immune system.

1 Halve the fennel lengthways, then slice very thinly into strips.

2 Spread the bread with olive or sun-dried tomato purée and top with the sliced peppers.

3 Mix together the dressing ingredients and season well.

4 Spoon over the peppers, cover with the other slices of bread to make sandwiches, and enjoy.

salads

fish salad with herb vinaigrette

Serves: 2

10 cherry tomatoes, halved
sea salt and freshly ground black pepper
1 tbsp extra-virgin olive oil
1 tsp balsamic vinegar
3 large handfuls of rocket
350 g hot smoked trout fillets
8 cooked large (or tiger) prawns, shelled
2 tbsp capers

for the dressing:
2 tbsp each chopped dill and chives,
sunflower oil, olive oil, and red wine vinegar
1 tsp Dijon mustard
pinch of sugar
freshly ground black pepper

Cherry tomatoes are good for **vitamin C**, a powerful antioxidant. Oil-rich fish, such as trout, provide **essential fats**, which are essential for a developing foetus, and prawns are a good source of **calcium**, **magnesium**, and **protein**. Prawns must be cooked thoroughly.

1 Preheat the oven to 180°C/ 350°F/gas mark 4. Put the cherry tomatoes in a roasting dish, season, and drizzle with oil. Roast for 10 minutes in the oven, then drizzle over the balsamic vinegar and roast for another 15 minutes, until lightly wilted. Leave to cool.
2 Make the dressing; put the ingredients into a screw-top jar,

replace the lid, and shake well until thick and emulsified.
3 Scatter the rocket over serving plates, top with the smoked trout and prawns, and scatter over with the capers and tomatoes. Drizzle over with the dressing and serve with hunks of fresh crusty bread.

new potato salad with bacon & avocado

Serves: 3

5 rashers back or streaky bacon
550 g new potatoes
handful of flat-leaf parsley, roughly chopped
2 carrots, washed or peeled and trimmed
2 celery sticks
1 avocado, peeled and stoned
large handful of watercress, roughly chopped
2 red peppers, deseeded and finely sliced
sea salt and freshly ground black pepper

for the vinaigrette dressing:
1½ tbsp lemon juice
3 tbsp extra-virgin olive oil
sea salt and freshly ground black pepper

Make this salad and eat for lunch on its own or for supper with a piece of grilled chicken or fish. Potatoes are very good **carbohydrates**, providing energy for the body. Carrots provide **betacarotene**, which is essential for good vision.

1 Preheat a grill and cook the bacon until crispy.
2 Cook the potatoes in boiling water for about 10–12 minutes, until tender when pierced with a knife. Drain and cut in half.
3 Make the dressing; whisk the lemon juice and oil together and season well. Pour the dressing over the warm potatoes in a salad bowl

(they will absorb the flavour from the dressing into their flesh). Add the parsley and mix everything together. Leave to stand for 10 minutes.
4 Thinly slice the carrots, celery, and avocado. Add the watercress and red pepper to the potatoes. Mix everything together, season to taste, and serve.

fennel & roast beet salad

Serves: 4

2 fennel bulbs
4 beetroots
1 tbsp balsamic vinegar
200 g mixed watercress,
rocket, and spinach
couple of handfuls each of sunflower and
pumpkin seeds, toasted

for the dressing:
1 tbsp balsamic
3 tbsp olive oil
1 large clove garlic, finely chopped
1-cm piece of fresh root ginger,
peeled and grated
sea salt and freshly
ground black pepper

If you want to make this slightly more substantial, serve with cottage cheese and bread.

Beetroot is a source of **folic acid**, which is very important in helping to prevent birth defects in the early stages of pregnancy. Mixed greens provide **betacarotene**, which helps to boost the immune system and the seeds are a great source of **essential fatty acids**.

1 Preheat the oven to 180°C/ 350°F/gas mark 6. Slice the fennel into thin wedges. Wrap the beets (with skin on) in foil parcels.
2 Arrange the beetroot in a roasting dish and roast in the oven for 30 minutes. Add the fennel and roast for another 10 minutes.
3 Drizzle the balsamic vinegar over the fennel and roast for another 10 minutes.

4 Slice the beets into wedges and put into a bowl. Add the fennel and mixed leaves.
5 Mix together the dressing ingredients. Drizzle the dressing over the salad and sprinkle over with the seeds.

"anything goes" salad with a honey & mint dressing

Serves: 3–4

handful of sunflower seeds
125 g baby spinach leaves, washed and sorted
handful of cherry tomatoes, quartered
handful of radishes, sliced
2 small beetroot, peeled and diced

for the dressing (this dressing makes enough for four):
handful of mint, finely chopped
1–2 cloves garlic, crushed
1 tsp runny honey
½–1 tsp Dijon mustard, to taste
sea salt and freshly ground black pepper
2 tbsp red-wine vinegar
4 tbsp extra-virgin olive oil

a couple of nice cheeses, e.g. Cornish Yarg and Red Leicester or smoked mackerel fillets, and fresh bread, to serve

Chose your favourite salad ingredients and add to the bowl – as long as you add some spinach. This is great served with smoked mackerel and fresh crusty bread.

There are quite a few benefits from the ingredients in this salad, depending on what you choose to throw in. To give you an idea: sunflower seeds contain **magnesium**, which is involved in producing energy; spinach is great for **iron**, which is essential to the development and growth of an unborn child; tomatoes are a good source of **vitamin C**, which assists in the absorption of iron; and beetroot is a good source of **folic acid**, which helps to reduce risks of spina bifida in the early stages of pregnancy.

1 Put the sunflower seeds into a dry frying pan and heat gently for a few minutes. Transfer to a large bowl and add all of the other salad ingredients.

2 Put the dressing ingredients into a screw-top jar, replace the lid, and shake well to mix. Pour the dressing over the salad, toss everything together, and serve with chunks of hard cheese or mackerel fillets and slices of fresh crusty bread.

cos, pear, & Parmesan salad

Serves: 3–4

100 g hazelnuts, chopped
2 small pears, peeled and cored
squeeze of lemon juice
2 heads of lettuce, washed and torn
100 g Parmesan cheese shavings

for the dressing:
3 tbsp extra-virgin olive oil
1 tbsp lemon juice
sea salt and freshly ground black pepper

Pears provide **fibre**, which helps with digestion. Hazelnuts are very high in **vitamin E**, which helps maintain healthy skin. Parmesan cheese provides **calcium**, which helps to prevent osteoporosis.

1 Dry-fry the hazelnuts in a frying pan, moving them around regularly until golden in colour.
2 Slice the pears into chunks and cover in lemon juice to prevent browning. Put into a bowl with the hazelnuts and lettuce.

3 Make the dressing; mix the oil and lemon juice together, and season. Pour the dressing over the salad and finish with fresh Parmesan shavings.

chickpea salad with cumin & yoghurt dressing

Serves: 4

½ cucumber
2 x 400 g cans chickpeas, drained
75 g sunblush tomatoes (available from Sainsbury's deli counter) or cherry tomatoes, finely chopped

for the dressing:
1 tsp cumin seeds, dry-fried and ground
2 tbsp natural yoghurt
handful of mint leaves, finely sliced
sea salt and freshly ground black pepper

This is quick and easy to make, and tastes fabulous. Cumin has quite a powerful flavour – add more or less to suit your taste.

Chickpeas provide **protein**, and cucumber is a source of **folic acid**, which is essential in the manufacture of **amino acids** and red blood cells.

Tomatoes are a good source of **vitamin C**, which strengthens the body's immune system.

1 Cut the cucumber in half lengthways, scoop out the seeds, and cut the flesh into small pieces or strips.
2 Put the chickpeas into a bowl and add the cucumber and sunblush or cherry tomatoes.

3 Mix together the dressing ingredients and pour over the salad. Toss everything together and serve.

soups

butternut squash & cumin soup

Serves: 6

1 tbsp olive oil
1 large onion, peeled and finely chopped
2 medium cloves garlic, peeled and chopped
½ tsp cumin seeds
½ tsp ground cumin
1 kg butternut squash, peeled & chopped into cubes
1.1 litres vegetable stock
1 tbsp tomato purée
freshly ground black pepper
a little semi-skimmed milk (optional)

Butternut squash is very high in **betacarotene**, which is essential for growth and a healthy immune system.

1 Heat the oil in a saucepan and sweat the onion until soft. Add the garlic, cumin seeds, and ground cumin, and cook for another minute.
2 Mix in the butternut squash, add the stock and tomato purée, and bring to the boil. Cover with a lid and simmer for 30 minutes, until the pumpkin is very soft.
3 Using a hand blender, purée the soup until smooth. Season with black pepper. If the mixture is too thick, thin it with some semi-skimmed milk.

pea soup

Serves: 6

1 tbsp olive oil, plus extra for drizzling
1 large onion, peeled and finely chopped
1 clove garlic, peeled and sliced
750 g frozen peas
1 litre vegetable stock
handful of mint leaves
75 g Parmesan cheese, freshly grated

Served with Parmesan, mint, and olive oil. This is the perfect soup for when you have no fresh vegetables in the house. Freeze any left over in plastic bags and heat through as and when needed.

Peas provide **protein**, helping the body in growth and development. They also contain **folic acid**, which can help to prevent birth defects.

1 Heat the oil in a large saucepan and sauté the onion and garlic. Add two-thirds of the peas, stock, and the mint, reserving some leaves for scattering. Cover and bring to the boil, then simmer for five minutes.
2 Purée the mixture in a food processor or blender. Return to the pan, add the remaining peas and stock, and simmer for five minutes.
3 Serve in warm soup bowls – spoon the Parmesan into the middle of each, scatter over the remaining mint leaves, and drizzle with olive oil.

Moroccan spiced lentil soup with prunes & apricots

Serves: 4

Lentils provide protein, which helps with growth and development. Prunes and apricots provide **fibre**, which aids the digestion process.

2 tbsp olive oil
5 carrots, peeled and chopped
2 celery sticks, chopped
2 onions, peeled and chopped
5 cloves garlic, peeled and chopped
1 tsp each cinnamon, allspice, and cumin
150 g green lentils
400 g can chopped tomatoes
200 ml fruity red wine
2 litres chicken stock
14 pieces mixed prunes and apricots
handful each of parsley and mint, chopped

1 Heat the oil in a large saucepan and sauté the carrots, celery, and onions for about five minutes. Add the garlic and sauté for another five minutes, until the vegetables begin to soften.

2 Add the spices and coat the vegetables, releasing their aroma.

3 Add the lentils, tomatoes, red wine, and stock. Bring to the boil and simmer, uncovered, for about 40 minutes, by which time the lentils should be cooked through.

4 Add the fruit and gently cook for another 10 minutes. Roughly purée in a food processor and stir in the herbs. If you like, serve it with a dollop of Greek yoghurt on top and fresh, crusty bread.

something hot

avocado & pepper tortilla pizzas

Makes: 3 pizzas

1 red pepper, halved and deseeded

1 large avocado

2–3 spring onions

1 red chilli, deseeded

3 flour tortillas

6 tbsp tomato purée

handful of cherry tomatoes, sliced

handful of black olives, stoned and sliced

75 g Cheddar cheese, finely grated

A very quick and easy way to eat a few more vegetables.

Flour tortillas make great pizza bases (as long as you like them thin and crispy), and they come in a multitude of flavours – for example, garlic and coriander. Try other toppings to suit your taste. Anchovies, pesto, mozzarella, tuna, and sweetcorn are all scrummy.

Red peppers and chillies are an excellent source of **vitamin C**, which is essential for growth and development. Avocados provide **vitamin E,** which helps to maintain healthy skin, and flour tortillas are a source of **carbohydrates**.

1 Thinly slice the red pepper. Cut the avocado in half and remove the stone. Peel and thinly slice the flesh. Thinly slice the spring onions and the chilli diagonally.

2 Spread each tortilla with one to two tablespoons tomato purée, scatter over with the pepper, avocado, tomatoes, spring onions, chilli, and olives, and top each with grated cheese.

3 Grill for three to five minutes, until the tortillas are crisp and golden and the cheese has melted.

other topping ideas

Thinly sliced tomatoes, wilted spinach, slices of grilled bacon, and grated Parmesan.

Tuna, anchovies, sliced and sautéed red onion, and lightly blanched broccoli.

Sliced tomatoes, crispy pancetta, grated cheese, olives, and finely chopped chilli or a sprinkling of chilli powder.

penne with an instant tomato sauce & herbs

Serves: 4

250 g penne or other pasta of your choice

250 g sunblush tomatoes (available from Sainsbury's deli counter)

1 clove garlic, peeled and roughly chopped

1 shallot, peeled and roughly chopped

sea salt and freshly ground black pepper

2 tsp aged balsamic vinegar (try and find a good one, but don't worry if you can't)

2 tbsp extra-virgin olive oil, plus extra for drizzling

6 basil leaves, chopped

bag of rocket leaves, to serve

Serve this pasta dish with a fresh green salad.

Pasta is a great **complex carbohydrate**, which provides slow-release energy to the body. Sunblush tomatoes contain **betacarotene** and **vitamin C**, both of which help boost the immune system.

1 Bring a pan of water to the boil. Add the pasta, and cook according to the instructions on the pack.

2 Blitz the remaining ingredients, except the basil and rocket, in a food processor for a few seconds, until the mixture resembles a chunky salsa. Mix with the cooked pasta.

3 Drizzle with a little extra olive oil and sprinkle with chopped basil. Serve hot or cold with the rocket leaves or any other green salad.

suppers
meat & poultry

chicken, chickpea, & sweet potato stew

Serves: 4

1 small organic chicken

5 cloves garlic

4 tbsp extra-virgin olive oil

sea salt and freshly ground black pepper

½ onion,

1 celery stick

1 bay leaf

a few peppercorns

4 leeks, trimmed and sliced

15 g sage leaves

2 tbsp lemon juice

2 sweet potatoes, peeled and chopped into small pieces

400 g can chickpeas, drained

olive oil, handful of fresh Parmesan cheese shavings, and crusty bread, to serve

This is delicious served in big bowls with chunks of fresh bread for mopping up the juices. If you do not have time to make your own stock, use Swiss Vegetable Bouillon Powder – it is by far the best bought stock. You could always roast a large chicken for supper one night and keep some of the meat to make this stew the next day.

Chicken is a very good source of **protein, minerals**, and **essential B vitamins**, all of which assist with growth and development. Chickpeas are a very good source of **protein** and **soluble fibre**, giving the body energy. Sweet potatoes are an excellent source of **betacarotene**, which strengthens the immune system.

1 Preheat the oven to 180°C/350°F/ gas mark 4. Put the chicken in a roasting tin, add the garlic cloves, drizzle with two tablespoons of the oil and season well. Roast for 40 minutes a kg plus an extra 10 minutes.

2 Carve the chicken meat, put the chicken carcass (without any skin) into a saucepan. Cover with cold water (approximately two pints), add half an onion and a stick of celery, a bay leaf and a few peppercorns, bring to the boil. Simmer for 20 minutes, strain.

3 Heat the remaining oil in a saucepan, add the leeks and sauté for five minutes. Add the soft roasted garlic, sage, lemon juice, chicken stock, sweet potato and chickpeas, simmer for 10 minutes, add enough chicken for four and cook for another five minutes or until all of the vegetables are cooked.

4 Serve with olive oil and Parmesan shavings on top and crusty bread for dipping.

Moroccan lamb with saffron and apricots

Serves: 6

large pinch of saffron threads (about 20)

4 tbsp olive oil

1.4 kg lamb fillet, cut into bite-size pieces

300 g button onions, peeled

3 cloves garlic, peeled and finely chopped

2 tbsp grated fresh root ginger

1½ tbsp ground coriander

2 tsp ground cumin, plus extra, to taste

large pinch of cayenne pepper

½ tsp cinnamon and 1 cinnamon stick

3 tsp harissa paste, plus extra, to taste

450 g crushed tomatoes (Rustica is best)

1 litre chicken stock

50 g each apricots, dates, and prunes

sea salt and freshly ground black pepper

25 g butter

50 g each almonds, pistachios, and dried cranberries

Serve with the Spicy Couscous with Roasted Vegetables, page 120, or with rice.

Lamb provides **protein** and **iron**, which are essential for a developing foetus. Tomatoes are a good source of **betacarotene** and **vitamin C**, which help boost the immune system.

1 Mix the saffron with one tablespoon of boiling water and let stand. Heat half the oil in a large frying pan and cook the lamb in batches for two to three minutes. Transfer to an ovenproof dish and keep warm.

2 Pour off all but one tablespoon of the oil from the pan, lower the heat, and cook the onions for five minutes, until golden. Stir in the saffron, garlic, ginger, spices, and harissa, and cook for one minute.

3 Add the tomatoes, stock, and fruit, bring to the boil, and season well. Stir in the lamb, cover and simmer, stirring occasionally, for 1½ hours, or until tender. Add the ground cumin and harissa to taste.

4 Heat the butter in a small saucepan, add the nuts and cranberries, and sauté for a couple of minutes. Spoon the lamb into a warm serving dish and scatter with the buttery nuts and fruit.

sautéed chicken breast with a mustard sauce

Serves: 4

1 tbsp butter
1 tbsp olive oil
4 chicken breasts
2 shallots, peeled and finely chopped
100 ml white wine
250 ml chicken stock
2 cloves garlic, finely chopped
170 ml whipping cream
1 tbsp wholegrain mustard
1 tbsp chopped tarragon
2 tsp finely chopped thyme
1 tbsp chopped parsley for scattering
sea salt and freshly ground black pepper

boiled potatoes or rice and
wilted spinach, to serve

The beauty of this dish is that it takes very little time to throw together and you can start to prepare it a little while before you need and then finish it off before serving.

Chicken is a good source of **protein**, which helps with growth and development. Whipping cream provides some **calcium**, helping to strengthen teeth and bones.

1 Heat the butter and the oil in a heavy-based frying pan over a medium-high heat. Add the chicken breasts and sauté for a few minutes on each side, until golden brown – this seals in the juices. Using a slotted spoon, transfer to a dish and keep warm.

2 Heat any oil and butter left in the pan, then add the shallots and sauté for one minute, until softened.

3 Add the wine, stock, and garlic, and bring to the boil. Boil until the liquid has reduced to about 125 ml.

4 Whisk in the cream and mustard and bring back to the boil. Cook until slightly thickened. Add the thyme, season to taste, and whisk thoroughly.

5 Return the chicken breasts to the pan and cook for five minutes, until cooked through but not overcooked. Scatter with fresh parsley and serve with potatoes or rice and wilted spinach.

Chinese-style honey-glazed duck with sweet & sticky pak choi

Serves: 4

4 duck breasts

1 tbsp Chinese five-spice powder

1 tbsp and 1 tsp honey

2 tsp soy sauce

400 g pak choi

1 tbsp olive oil

1 red chilli, deseeded and finely chopped

2 cloves garlic, peeled and finely chopped

1 tbsp finely chopped fresh root ginger

1 tbsp hoisin

1 tbsp mirin

Pak choi can be green- or white-stemmed and it comes in many shapes and sizes. Mirin is a form of sweetened sake, which is available from good supermarkets.

Chicken is a very good source of **protein** and **minerals**, which are vital for growth and development. Pak choi is a good source of **betacarotene** and **vitamin C**, which both strengthen the immune system. Ginger is thought to relieve morning sickness.

1 Preheat the oven to 200°C/ 400°F/gas mark 6. Heat a heavy-based frying pan, add the duck breasts, and sear skin-side down for a few minutes, until brown – you do not need to add any extra oil to the pan.

2 Mix together the five-spice powder, one tablespoon of the honey, and one tablespoon of the soy sauce, and brush liberally all over the duck breasts. Put onto a baking tray and roast in the oven for eight minutes – the meat should still be slightly springy to the touch. Leave to rest.

3 Bring a little water to the boil in a saucepan, add the pak choi, and cook for few minutes, until wilted but still slightly crisp in texture.

4 Heat the oil in a frying pan, add the chilli, garlic, and ginger, and sauté for a couple of minutes. Add the hoisin, mirin, and the remaining soy sauce and honey. Cook for one minute, then drizzle over the pak choi. Slice the duck and serve with the pak choi.

fish

plaice with a Sicilian stuffing

Serves: 4

4 large plaice fillets, skinned and halved

1–2 tbsp olive oil

for the filling:

2 tbsp each fresh white breadcrumbs and extra-virgin olive oil

1 tbsp shredded basil leaves

2 tsp each finely chopped mint and chopped capers

1 tbsp each pine nuts, raisins, and chopped olives

Serve with roasted red peppers, spinach, and a balsamic vinaigrette. Fish and nuts are good sources of protein, which helps with the baby's growth and development. The nuts provide a good source of fat. serve thefish with roasted red peppers, spinach and a balsamic vinaigrette.

1 Preheat the oven to 200°C/ 400°F/gas mark 6. Mix all the filling ingredients together. Spoon a teaspoon of the filling on top of each fillet half at the wider end, and roll up.

2 Pack tightly into an ovenproof dish, scatter over any extra stuffing, and drizzle with oil. Bake in the oven for about eight minutes, depending on the size of the fish, until cooked through.

oven-baked lemon & herb risotto with monkfish rosemary skewers

Serves: 4

25 g butter

2 tbsp olive oil

1 onion or 3 shallots, finely chopped

175 g arborio rice

100 ml white wine

675 ml light vegetable stock

zest of 1 lemon

600 g monkfish tail, cubed

rosemary sprigs for skewering

2 tbsp extra-virgin olive oil

50 g Parmesan cheese, grated

4 tbsp chopped basil

sea salt and freshly ground black pepper

1 lemon, cut into chunks, to serve

A much less time-consuming way of preparing risotto is to throw it into the oven rather than standing over the stove stirring. There is only a small amount of wine added and the alcohol content is minimal.

1 Preheat the oven to 180°C/ 350°F/gas mark 4.
2 Melt the butter and oil in a heavy-based pan and fry the onion or shallots slowly, without colouring, for five to 10 minutes, until softened. Turn the heat up slightly, add the rice to the pan, and stir, thoroughly coating with the buttery onion. Stir for a minute or two to coat the grains.
3 Add the wine and let that bubble. Add the stock and bring up to simmering point. Stir once and transfer to a warm ovenproof dish. Put in the middle of the oven,

uncovered. After 20 minutes, remove from the oven, stir once, and add the lemon zest. Return to the oven for 15 minutes.
4 Carefully skewer the fish on to the rosemary and brush with oil. Cook under a hot grill for two to three minutes on each side, until cooked through. Cover the ends of the rosemary with foil to prevent burning.
5 When the risotto is ready, stir in the Parmesan and basil. Season well and leave to stand for a couple of minutes before serving with the fish and chunks of lemon.

Goan fish curry with chickpea, lemon, & spinach rice

Serves: 4

Fish and rice are both good sources of **protein**, which is essential for a developing foetus. Creamed coconut provides some **calcium**, which helps to strengthen teeth and bones, and ginger is thought to be good for relieving morning sickness. Spinach is a good source of **folic acid**, which helps to reduce birth defects during early pregnancy.

for the rice:

300 ml basmati rice

zest of 1 lemon

410 g can chickpeas, drained and rinsed

200 g baby spinach

sea salt and freshly ground black pepper

for the fish curry:

2 tbsp vegetable oil

2 onions, peeled and chopped

large piece of fresh root ginger, peeled and chopped

3 cloves garlic, peeled and chopped

2 stalks lemon grass, crushed with a rolling pin

2 red chillies, deseeded and finely chopped

3 tsp turmeric

6 cardamom pods

2 tsp garam masala

2–3 tsp medium curry powder

500 g mixed fresh fish, e.g. monkfish, salmon, and raw tiger prawns

100 g creamed coconut, cut into pieces

1 Put the rice, lemon zest, and 600 ml water in a saucepan, cover, and bring to the boil.
2 Reduce the heat and simmer, still covered, for exactly 14 minutes. Remove from the heat and quickly add the chickpeas. Cover and leave to stand for exactly nine minutes. Remove the lid and add the spinach. Cover and let stand for another couple of minutes.
3 Make the curry: heat the oil in a saucepan, add the onion, ginger, garlic, lemon grass, and chillies, and cook for 10 minutes. Stir constantly without letting the onions brown. Add the turmeric, cardamom pods, garam masala, and curry powder. Mix well and cook for another five minutes.
4 Cut the fish into large chunks, add to spice mix along with 75 ml water, and simmer for five minutes. Add the prawns and cook for another five minutes.
5 Add the creamed coconut and stir carefully until it has melted – it should not boil. Serve with the chickpea and spinach rice.

fennel & citrus fruit salmon

Serves: 4

700 g new potatoes, scrubbed and cut into small pieces

1 tbsp fennel seeds, roasted and crushed

zest of 1 lime and 1 lemon

40 g fresh breadcrumbs

4 salmon fillets

sea salt and freshly ground black pepper

1–2 tbsp olive oil

1–2 tsp Dijon mustard

200 g sugar snap peas

1 lemon, cut into wedges, to serve

The salmon has a subtle but delicious crunchy topping. Serve with potatoes and green vegetables.

Potatoes provide **carbohydrate**, for slow-releasing energy. Salmon is a good source of **protein** and **essential fatty acids**, which are vital for growth and development. Sugar snaps are a good source of **vitamin C**, strengthening the immune system.

1 Preheat the oven to 200°C/ 400°F/gas mark 6. Bring a pan of water to the boil, add the potatoes, and cook until tender. Mix together the fennel seeds, lime and lemon zests, and breadcrumbs.

2 Season the salmon fillets with salt and pepper. Heat the oil in a heavy-based pan and sauté the salmon (skin side up) for 30–40 seconds, moving constantly so that they do not stick. Turn over and sauté for another 30 seconds, moving around in the pan. Remove from the heat, brush the salmon with the mustard, and sprinkle over a layer of the crumb mixture, packing it onto the salmon. Place the pan on the top shelf of the oven and cook for four to five minutes until cooked through.

3 Meanwhile, blanch the sugar snap peas in boiling water for a minute. Remove the fish from the oven and let rest for a few minutes before serving with lemon wedges, the boiled potatoes and sugar snap peas.

spiced lentils with prawns

Serves: 4

190 g Puy lentils

375 ml water

2 spring onions, finely sliced

2 tbsp extra-virgin olive oil

2 tbsp red-wine vinegar

1 red chilli, seeded, finely chopped

sea salt and freshly ground black pepper

1 tsp each ground coriander, ground cumin, and turmeric

½ cup coriander leaves, chopped

20 raw prawns, shelled

100 g green beans

150 g baby spinach leaves

handful of mint leaves

for the dressing:

75 ml natural yoghurt

2 tbsp lime juice

4 tbsp chopped mint

This is incredibly tasty, low in fat, and packed with nutrients.

Lentils and prawns are a good source of **protein**, which is important for growth and development. Prawns must be cooked thoroughly.

1 Place the lentils and water in a medium saucepan and bring to the boil. Reduce the heat and simmer for 15 minutes. Drain the lentils.

2 Put the warm lentils, spring onions, one tablespoon of the olive oil, vinegar, chilli, salt and pepper, ground coriander, cumin, ½ tsp of the turmeric and half the fresh coriander in a bowl, stir to combine, and set aside.

3 Put the remaining oil, turmeric, fresh coriander, and seasoning in a bowl and stir to combine. Add the prawns and stir to coat.

4 Heat a non-stick frying pan, add the prawns, and cook for a couple of minutes, until they turn pink all over, shaking the pan frequently.

5 Bring a little water in a saucepan to the boil, add the green beans, and blanch for a couple of minutes, then add the spinach and let it wilt for a minute.

6 To serve, divide the lentils among four plates, top with the beans, spinach, mint, and prawns. Mix together the dressing ingredients and drizzle over the salad.

vegetarian

spicy couscous with roasted vegetables

Serves: 6

2 each red and yellow peppers, deseeded

2 medium aubergines

8 ripe tomatoes, halved

6 cloves garlic, peeled

2 red onions, peeled and sliced into thin wedges

2 tbsp olive oil

sea salt and freshly ground black pepper

500 g couscous

750 ml boiling vegetable stock
(or enough to cover couscous)

large knob butter

1 tsp crushed dried red chilli

2–3 tsp harissa paste

for the chermoula:

1 tsp each fennel and cumin seeds, toasted and ground

50 g each coriander and mint, roughly chopped

125 g parsley, roughly chopped

3 tsp paprika

large pinch of cayenne

pinch of salt

3 cloves garlic, peeled and roughly chopped

zest of 1 orange

250 ml olive oil

The chermoula gives the couscous a wonderful flavour. However, if you are short of time, omit the chermoula and serve the couscous with roasted vegetables – it is still a great dish.

Couscous is a **complex carbohydrate,** providing energy to the body. Peppers, tomatoes, and aubergines are all sources of **vitamin C**, which provides natural immunity.

1 Preheat the oven to 200°C/400°F/gas mark 6. Cut the peppers into chunks and slice the aubergines. Arrange all the vegetables in a roasting tin, pour over the oil, and toss around until coated. Season, and roast in the oven for 35–45 minutes, turning once, until cooked and golden at the edges.

2 Put the couscous into an ovenproof dish, cover the grains with boiling stock, and leave for 10 minutes for the grains to swell. Dot the butter over the top, season, and sprinkle with the chilli. Cover with foil and bake alongside the vegetables for 25 minutes.

3 Meanwhile, make the chermoula: put all the ingredients into a food processor and whiz until smooth. Add the harissa, roasted vegetables, and three to four tablespoons of the chermoula to the couscous. Mix everything together and serve.

NB: serve any left over chermoula with grilled fish for a quick supper.

squash & thyme tarts with relish

Serves: 6

This makes a perfect supper served with a fresh watercress salad.

for the filling:
450 g squash, halved and deseeded
1 tbsp olive oil and 25 g butter
1 small leek, trimmed and chopped
2 cloves garlic
1 egg
40 g Parmesan cheese, grated
90 ml double cream
45 ml milk
fresh thyme plus extra sprigs for serving

for the pastry:
180 g plain flour
pinch of salt
1 tsp finely chopped thyme
90 g unsalted butter, cut into
small pieces and chilled
1 egg
ice-cold water

for the beetroot and red onion relish:
2 chopped red onions, caramelized
1 cooked beetroot, finely chopped
1 tbsp balsamic vinegar

1 Preheat the oven to 200°C/ 400°F/gas mark 6. Roast the squash for 40 minutes, until soft.
2 Make the pastry: sift the flour and salt into a food processor, add the thyme, and pulse for a few seconds. Add the butter and process to make fine breadcrumbs. Keeping the machine running, add the egg and a little water if necessary, 1 tbsp at a time. If the pastry is still in crumbly pieces, add a little more water. To make by hand, sift the flour into a large bowl with the salt. Add the chopped butter and rub the fat into the flour. Stir in the thyme. Add water a little at a time and bring together to form a ball. Wrap in cling film and chill for at least 30 minutes.
3 Roll out the pastry and line four 10-cm tart tins. Chill for 30 minutes.

4 Lower the oven to 180°C/ 350°F/gas mark 4. Heat a baking tray until hot. Cover the pastry with sheets of baking paper and baking beans, place the tins on the tray, and bake for 10 minutes. Remove the paper and beans, and cook for another five minutes.
5 Heat the oil and butter in a small saucepan, add the leek and garlic, and sauté for a few minutes, until soft. Scoop out the cooked squash flesh and put in a food processor with the egg, ¾ of the cheese, cream, milk, and thyme. Process until smooth (or mix well by hand).
6 Fill the tart cases with the squash mixture, top with the remaining cheese. Bake for about 20 minutes, until slightly puffed and golden. Mix together the ingredients for the beetroot and red onion relish and serve with the tarts.

Thai-style curry with tofu

Serves: 4

25 ml sesame oil

2 red onions, finely sliced

3 cloves garlic, peeled and finely chopped

2 red chillies, deseeded and finely sliced (with a few seeds for a little kick), plus a little chilli powder

4-cm piece of fresh root ginger, peeled and finely chopped

2 tbsp tomato purée

1 stalk lemon grass, crushed with a rolling pin

lime leaves or zest of 1 lime

400 g soft tofu, cut into small pieces

200 g sugar snap peas, sliced

300 ml coconut milk

200 ml vegetable stock

2-3 tsp fish sauce

3–4 large handfuls of baby spinach leaves

large handful each of coriander leaves and cashew nuts, chopped and toasted, or sesame seeds or pumpkin seeds, toasted

Tofu is the Japanese name given to soya bean curd and is a very good vegetarian source of **protein**, **calcium**, and **iron**, which is essential for a developing foetus. It has the added advantage of being low in saturated fat, contains no cholesterol, and has almost no sodium. Spinach is a good source of **folic acid**, **betacarotene**, and **iron**. Coconut milk also provides some **calcium**, aiding in the development of strong teeth and bones. Ginger is thought to be very good for relieving morning sickness.

1 Heat the oil in a frying pan or wok. Add the onions and fry, stirring well, until deeply coloured. Add the garlic, chillies, and ginger, and fry for another minute, stirring all the time.
2 Add the tomato purée, lemon grass, lime leaves or lime zest, tofu, and sugar snap peas, and stir gently over a medium heat for a minute, to coat the tofu.

3 Add the coconut milk, stock, and fish sauce, and simmer, uncovered, for four minutes. Add the spinach and toss together. Cook for another two minutes. Serve with lots of fresh coriander, and cashew nuts or seeds scattered over the top.

orange peppers with a brioche filling

Serves: 4

2 orange peppers

2 yellow peppers

75 g brioche crumbs
(about 3–4 thick slices)

2 tbsp pine nuts, toasted and
roughly chopped

handful each of flat-leaf parsley and mint

250 g haloumi cheese

handful of black olives, stoned (optional)

zest of 1 orange

2 tbsp extra-virgin olive oil

sea salt and freshly ground black pepper

Brioche is a fabulous sweet, rich bread which makes wonderful crumbs ideal for stuffing roasted peppers.

Haloumi cheese is a very good source of **protein** and **calcium**, which are important for growth and development of strong teeth and bones. Peppers are an excellent source of **vitamin C**, which boosts the immune system. Pine nuts are a very good source of **magnesium** and **zinc**, which are both important for growth.

1 Preheat the oven to 190°C/ 375°F/gas mark 5. Put the whole peppers in a roasting tin and roast for 45 minutes, until soft.

2 Put the brioche crumbs onto a baking sheet and toast in the oven for five minutes, turning the crumbs now and then until golden and crisp. Put into a bowl. Add the pine nuts, herbs, cheese, olives, zest, and half the oil to the crumbs, mix together, and season to taste.

3 Remove the stalks from the peppers and scoop out the seeds. Fill the peppers with the crumb mixture and drizzle over the remaining oil. Bake for 15 minutes, until warmed through.

desserts

coconut & cardamom rice pudding

Serves: 4

3 cardamom pods
150 g pudding rice
250 ml full-fat or semi-skimmed milk
250 ml coconut milk
100 ml water
few drops of vanilla extract
25 g golden caster sugar

The rice is a good source of **carbohydrates**, providing slow-release energy. It is therefore a great pudding to eat at lunchtime.

1 Spilt the cardamom pods in half, put the seeds into a mortar and crush with a pestle.
2 Put the rice, milk, coconut milk, water, vanilla, and crushed cardamom seeds into a saucepan. Bring to the boil, then reduce the heat and simmer for about 15–20 minutes, stirring frequently to

prevent it from sticking to the bottom. If necessary, add a few tablespoons of water to loosen the mixture.
3 Add the sugar, mix well, and cook for a minute. Serve on its own or with fresh fruit.

little cherry & almond puddings

Makes: 4

for the caramel:
75 g butter
50 g sugar
1 tbsp water
225 g cherries, stoned, plus extra for serving

for the sponge:
90 g softened butter
90 g golden caster sugar
50 g plain flour
50 g ground almonds
1 tsp baking powder

thick Greek yoghurt, to serve

Serve the puddings with some fresh cherries alongside. Cherries are a great source of **magnesium** and **potassium**.

1 Preheat the oven to 190°C/ 375°F/gas mark 5.
2 Make the caramel; melt the butter, sugar, and water together and leave to bubble until golden brown.
3 Butter four small pudding moulds or ramekins and divide the stoned cherries among them. Pour over with the caramel.
4 Make the sponge; beat together the butter and sugar. Gradually add the flour, ground almonds and baking powder. Quickly beat again to mix. Spoon this batter over the cherries.

5 Put the tins onto a tray and bake in the oven for about 30 minutes, until golden and springy to the touch. Let stand for a few minutes, run a knife around the edge of the moulds or ramekins, and unmould onto a plate. Serve with a dollop of thick Greek yoghurt and some extra cherries.

lemon & poppy seed slice with crushed berry sauce

Serves: 6–8

225 g each cottage cheese
and cream cheese
175 ml sour cream
150 g golden caster sugar
juice of 1 lemon
grated zest of 2 lemons
2 tbsp cornflour
3 organic eggs
1 tbsp poppy seeds

for the sauce:
250 g raspberries
50 g caster sugar
juice of ½ lemon

The cheeses are great a source of **calcium,** and the fresh raspberries also provide **calcium,** along with **potassium, iron,** and **magnesium.** Raspberries retain their flavour better if they are unwashed, so it is best to choose organic.

1 Preheat the oven to 150°C/ 300°F/gas mark 2. Butter and line a 23-cm springform flan tin.
2 Put the cheeses, sour cream, sugar, lemon juice and zest, and cornflour into a food processor and whiz until smooth. Whiz in the eggs one at a time, then stir in the poppy seeds.

3 Pour the mixture into the prepared tin and bake in the oven for about one hour, until just set and slightly puffed. Run a knife around the edge to prevent splitting as it cools.
4 Put the ingredients for the raspberry sauce into a food processor and whiz together. Serve in slices with the sauce drizzled over the top.

snacks
things on bruschetta

bruschetta

Take a part-baked ciabatta loaf and cook according to the pack instructions. Slice thickly and arrange on a baking tray. Drizzle with oil and return to the hot oven for a few minutes until crisp and golden. Turn over and cook for a few minutes on the other side. Rub each side with garlic. Munch on these with one of the following toppings.

sardines with lemon & pepper

2 ripe tomatoes, sliced

120 g can sardines in olive oil, drained and oil reserved

freshly ground black pepper

squeeze of lemon

Sardines contain **essential fatty acids**, which are very important for healthy eyes and brain function, especially in unborn babies. Bread is a good source of **fibre**, which helps with digestion. Tomatoes are very rich in **vitamin C**, which is essential for growth.

1 Lay the tomato slices on top of the toasted ciabatta. Arrange the sardines close to each other on the tomatoes, breaking them up slightly with the back of a fork.

Season with pepper and lemon juice.
2 Drizzle with a little olive oil from the sardine can, put under a hot grill for a minute, and serve.

smashed cannellini beans with lemon

175 g can cannellini beans, drained and rinsed

1 clove garlic, peeled and crushed

zest and juice of ½–1 lemon

2–3 tbsp extra-virgin olive oil, 6 basil leaves

2 tbsp freshly grated Parmesan cheese

Beans are a great source of **fibre** and **protein**.

1 Mash all the ingredients, except the Parmesan, in a bowl, or whiz in a food processor or blender.

2 Season with sea salt and black pepper and spread onto the toasted ciabatta. Top with Parmesan to serve.

avocado, coriander, & lime

1 avocado
handful of coriander leaves
juice of ½ lime

Avocados are a good source of **potassium** and **vitamins E** and **A**.

1 Cut the avocado in half and remove the stone. Peel and slice the flesh into strips.

2 Arrange the avocado strips on the ciabatta, scatter over the coriander, and drizzle with lime juice.

artichoke, lemon, & Parmesan

jar of artichokes hearts in oil, drained
squeeze of lemon juice
freshly ground black pepper
2 tbsp finely grated Parmesan cheese
dark-green salad leaves

Artichokes supply both **phosphorus** and **iron**, and are also good for the digestion.

1 Lightly mash the artichokes, add the lemon juice and pepper, and spoon onto the ciabatta.

2 Top with the Parmesan. Eat with a handful of fresh green salad leaves.

super quick snacks

carrot hummus

400 g can chickpeas, drained and rinsed

3 medium carrots, peeled and chopped

2 tbsp tahini (roasted sesame seed paste)

juice of ½–1 lime or lemon

50 ml water

3 tbsp olive oil

2 cloves garlic, peeled and crushed

sea salt and freshly ground black pepper

a selection of vegetables, e.g. baby carrots, celery, baby tomatoes, and radishes, and pitta chips, to serve

This will last for a few days in the fridge.

1 Put all the ingredients into a food processor and blend until smooth. Adjust the seasoning to taste.

2 Make the pitta chips; cut the pitta bread in half lengthways, then cut each half into little triangles and toast under a medium grill for a few minutes, until golden and crisp.

3 Serve the hummus with crudités and/or pitta chips.

roasted pumpkin seeds

bag of pumpkin seeds

2 tsps paprika

good drizzle of olive oil

sea salt and freshly ground black pepper

Pumpkin are particularly favoured for their high **zinc**, **calcium**, **B vitamins**, and **essential fatty acid** levels. Eaten regularly, pumpkin seeds can rid the intestinal tract of unwanted parasites.

1 Preheat the oven to 190°C/ 375°F/gas mark 5. Spread the pumpkin seeds on a baking tray and sprinkle with the paprika.

2 Drizzle with oil, season well, and roast in the oven for 10 minutes, turning occasionally. Leave to cool, then store in an airtight container.

nuts & bolts

1 tsp of each cumin seeds, coriander seeds, paprika & black pepper

200 g crunchy cereal of your choice, e.g. toasted muesli or granola

1 tbsp each cashew nuts, hazelnuts, pumpkin seeds, sunflower seeds

1 tbsp of each dried cranberries, dried, chopped apricots

1-2 tbsp olive oil for drizzling

This is a fun, crunchy snack to munch on. Use any cereal that you fancy and add spices of your choice,such as Chinese five spice.

1 Preheat the oven to 180°C/350°F/gas mark 4. Heat the spices in a dry frying pan to toast lightly. Crush with a pestle and mortar.
2 Spread the cereal, spices, nuts, and fruit onto a baking tray. Drizzle with the oil and toss well to coat.
3 Roast in the oven for 15–20 minutes, turning frequently. Leave to cool, store in an airtight container.

fresh ginger tea

Serves: 4–5

900 ml water

3 cardamom pods

1 cinnamon stick

5-cm piece of fresh root ginger, peeled and freshly grated

ice cubes and fresh fruit, e.g. apple and orange slices, to serve (optional)

Try this tea if you are suffering from morning sickness – it may help to relieve some of the symptoms. If you are serving the tea cold, you could always add a few pieces of freshly sliced fruit.

1 Put the water in a saucepan and add the remaining ingredients. Bring to the boil and leave to simmer for three minutes to allow the spices to infuse.
2 Strain the tea and serve hot or chilled with ice cubes and slices of fresh fruit.

breads & cakes

coconut and fruit bread

(toddler-friendly if child is tolerant of seeds)

Makes: one 1-kg loaf

Coconut, milk, and natural yoghurt all contain **calcium**, which helps to strengthen bones and teeth. Dried fruit is a very good source of **fibre**, which helps with digestion.

2 eggs

200 ml milk

100 ml natural yoghurt

few drops vanilla extract

275 g plain flour

2 tsp each baking powder and ground cinnamon

195 g golden caster sugar

100 g desiccated coconut

100 g mixed dried fruit, e.g cranberries, cherries, apricots, and pineapple, chopped

30 g sunflower seeds, plus extra for sprinkling

50 g butter, melted

1 Preheat the oven to 180°C/ 350°F/gas mark 4. Grease and lightly flour a 1-kg loaf tin. Gently whisk together the eggs, milk, yoghurt, and vanilla.
2 Sift the flour, baking powder, and cinnamon into a bowl, add the sugar, coconut, fruit, and sunflower seeds, and stir to combine. Make a well in the centre and gradually stir in the egg mixture until just combined. Add the melted butter and stir until just smooth, being careful not to over-mix.
3 Pour into the prepared tin, sprinkle with sunflower seeds, and bake for 50 minutes to one hour, until a skewer inserted comes out clean. Leave in the tin for five minutes, then remove to a wire rack and leave to cool.

banana, fig, and honey cake

(toddler-friendly if child is tolerant of seeds)

Makes: one 20-cm cake

3 medium eggs

175 g soft brown sugar

200 ml sunflower oil

175 ml milk

125 g plain flour

125 g wholemeal flour

½ tsp bicarbonate soda

1 tsp ground cinnamon

large pinch of nutmeg

1 tsp ground mixed spice

2 bananas, peeled and mashed

250 g dried figs or dates, stoned and chopped

3 tbsps runny honey

This cake is very easy to make and will keep in an airtight tin; alternatively, cut in pieces and put in the freezer. If you feel the urge for a piece of naughty cream-filled cake, eat a piece of this instead.

Bananas are an excellent source of **potassium** and **fibre**, which help with the normal functioning of cells and digestion. They are also very good for energy. Figs, dates, and wholemeal flour all provide **fibre**, which helps with the digestion process.

1 Preheat the oven to 190°C/ 375°F/gas mark 5. Butter and flour a 20-cm cake tin.

2 Put everything into a bowl, except the bananas, figs or dates, and honey, and whisk until mixed together. Stir in the mashed bananas and chopped figs or dates.

3 Spoon into the prepared tin and bake in the oven for 45 minutes to one hour, until a skewer inserted comes out clean. Make holes over the cake with a fork and pour over the honey.

fruity nutty bread

Makes: one 1-kg loaf

2 tbsp sunflower oil

350 g plain flour

150 g wholemeal flour

1 tsp sea salt

1 tsp cream of tartar

1 tsp baking soda

1 tsp baking powder

100 g each mixed nuts, toasted and roughly chopped, sunflower seeds, plus extra for sprinkling, and dried apricots, roughly chopped

250 ml natural yoghurt

25 ml milk

honey

This is a very quick "yeast-free" bread. It is delicious cut into slices and served with a really fruity jam or mashed banana and cinnamon.

1 Preheat the oven to 180°C/ 350°F/gas mark 4. Grease a 1-kg loaf tin with half the oil. Sieve the flours, salt, cream of tartar, baking soda, and baking powder together in a large bowl. Stir in the nuts, sunflower seeds, and apricots.

2 Mix together the yoghurt, milk, honey, and remaining oil. Stir this yoghurt mixture into the dry ingredients and mix to form a soft

dough. Spoon the batter into the oiled tin. Sprinkle sunflower seeds over the top.

3 Bake in the oven for one hour – you may need to cover the loaf with greaseproof paper after 40 minutes to prevent it from going too brown.

breastfeeding diet

breast feeding care

Put simply, breast milk provides all the essential nutrients a baby needs for best possible development. There is no substitute.

advantages

Some mothers decide that they don't want to try breastfeeding, and instead bottle-feed their babies from birth. Studies show that half of all UK mothers are breastfeeding their babies two weeks after birth, and only just over a quarter are still breastfeeding their babies at four months.

In the UK, a government campaign is under way to try to change this, and to encourage more mothers to breastfeed. When you look at the list of advantages to both the baby and the mother, you can see why it is so important.

Put simply, breast milk provides all the essential nutrients a baby needs for best possible development. There is no substitute. Of course, some mothers do have problems with breastfeeding, but for those who are able to make the choice, breast is certainly best.

The British Department of Health recommends that "mothers should be encouraged and supported in breastfeeding for at least four months and may choose to continue to breastfeed as the weaning diet becomes increasingly varied."

breastfeeding benefits

- You can usually begin to breastfeed your baby within an hour after birth. The first milk that a mother produces is called colostrum – a yellowish transparent fluid – which is usually excreted for the first three days. It contains less fat, more protein, and more protective factors than the breast milk that is produced later on. These protective factors can help fight polio, mumps, and *E. coli.*
- Colostrum also contains a high concentration of zinc, which is essential for a child's growth and development.
- Breastfeeding just after the birth also prompts your pituitary gland to release oxytocin, the hormone that causes the uterus to contract and expel the placenta soon after birth, helping to keep bleeding to a minimum.
- Studies show that breastfed babies have higher IQs than bottle-fed babies because of the essential fatty acids and other key nutrients in breast milk, despite the genetic make-up of the parents.
- A baby's digestive system is far from fully developed in the first few weeks, so the mother's milk is designed to meet its digestive and nutritional needs. As the baby and its needs develop, so does the mother's milk. Even when the baby's system is strong enough to accept solids, human milk is recommended as the main nutritional source until the baby is one year old. Human milk continues to boost the immune system for as long as it is offered. It takes between two and six years for a child's digestive system to reach full maturity (*Ref. 5.1*).
- Breast milk contains special proteins, antibodies, and white blood cells which help to protect the baby against infection and disease. Infant formulas don't contain such properties. As a result, bowel and lung infections tend to be more common in bottle-fed babies. breastfeeding may also help prevent diarrhoea and urinary-tract infections in babies. There is also evidence to show that the incidence of ear infections is significantly reduced in babies who breastfeed for longer than four months.
- It is nearly impossible for a baby to become allergic to its mother's milk.
- Breastfeeding may prevent milk- and other food-related allergies. There are more than 20 substances in cow's milk shown to be human allergens (*Ref. 5.2*). Colic and vomiting are often caused by cow's-milk allergy.
- Breastfeeding can help protect against allergies in babies in two ways. Firstly, breastfed babies are exposed to fewer allergens in the first months of life. Secondly, babies' immune systems are immature. They have previously relied on antibodies from their mothers while in the womb. Now that they are born, their systems are most suited to their mother's milk.
- Breast milk is convenient, cheap, and easy for most mothers.
- It is especially important for our baby to breastfeed for as long as possible if he or she is not being vaccinated, since breast milk helps to build the immune system and protect against disease.

breastfeeding disadvantages

There are very few disadvantages to breastfeeding.

● The only disadvantage that I found while breastfeeding my daughter Ella was that I had to be available at all times, which was fine until I needed to start working again. However, there are ways to cope with this. For further information, contact the National Chlidbirth Trust (NCT) or La Leche League (see "Useful Addresses", page 143).

● Some mothers may find it frustrating to watch what they eat for another few months after being "careful" for the last 40 (or longer) weeks. But remember that it is not difficult to eat a good, varied diet, and it is important in any case that you eat well for your own health as well as that of your baby.

● It is often hard to tell how much milk the baby is drinking from the breast, whereas the quantity of bottle milk can be regulated very easily. However, it is said to be impossible to over-feed a breastfed baby.

why organic breast is best

Organic breast milk is best. The longer a mother has been eating organically and reducing her exposure to environmental toxins, the better. Some studies have shown that pesticide residues and other harmful by-products of intensive farming can be passed to babies through breast milk.

In June 1999, this was documented in "Chemical Trespass", a World Wildlife Fund UK research report, which stated that babies were ingesting up to 42 times the World Health Organization (WHO) tolerable daily intake of dioxin-like compounds through breast milk.

Examples of chemicals found in breast milk in the UK include dioxins, toxic metals, and pesticides, all of which may have a variety of harmful effects to the baby. According to the British Ministry of Agriculture, Fisheries, and Food (MAFF), the primary source of dioxins in the UK are milk and dairy products, fish and fish oils, and animal and meat fats. A study carried out by MAFF reported that food, food packaging, and goods such as cleaning agents, cosmetics, and sunscreens are the main causes of contamination.

disadvantages of cow's milk

Calves have different development and growth needs to that of human babies. Cow's milk is geared to meet a calf's needs. A calf's body grows extremely rapidly and doesn't have the need to develop a highly complex brain.

There is also a school of thought which maintains that pasteurising cow's milk makes it difficult to digest and destroys useful enzymes (Ref. 5.3).

breast milk & nutrition

There are many advantages to eating a well-balanced diet. This is particularly true when breastfeeding. You will feel better, be more resistant to illness, and have more energy to cope with the new changes in your life.

However, for women who worry about the days they didn't eat as well as they could have, the following research should help put minds at rest.

According to UK National Childbirth Trust breastfeeding counsellor Heather Welford, "Your breast milk provides all the food and drink your baby needs, but do take care of yourself, too. Eat according to your hunger to maintain your energy levels."

The American National Academy of Sciences Subcommittee on Lactation confirmed this in its 1991 summary "Nutrition During Lactation". "Women living under a wide variety of circumstances in the US and elsewhere are capable of fully nourishing their infants by breastfeeding them. Mothers are able to produce milk of sufficient quantity and quality to support growth and promote the health of infants – even when the mother's supply of nutrients and energy is limited."

Even with a less-than-ideal diet, a mother's milk is the perfect food for her baby. Studies conducted in developing nations indicate that even "mild malnutrition appears to have only a slight effect, if any, on milk output", and no effect on the composition of mother's milk. As Ruth Lawrence, MD, writes: "All over the world, women produce adequate and even abundant milk on very inadequate diets (*Ref. 5.4*)."

There are no complicated "diet rules" to follow and, contrary to popular belief, there are few foods that must be avoided by nursing mothers. If you are already eating a healthy diet, there is no reason to change while you are breastfeeding.

Most breastfeeding mothers find that they can eat what they like without their diets having any adverse effects on their babies. Occasionally, however – especially in families with a history of food allergy – a food in the mother's diet does affect her nursing baby. Some babies can be affected after their mothers have eaten something particularly strong or spicy, or when they have an unusually large amount of a particular food or drink.

foods to avoid

The most common offenders are foods such as chocolate, dairy products, wheat, and soya products. If the baby seems to be upset by a particular food or drink avoid it and continue breastfeeding – everything should be back to normal within a day or so. For more information about healthy eating guidelines, *see* pages 34–61.

The key to successful breastfeeding is plenty of rest, a varied diet of small, frequent meals, lots of water – drink at least two litres a day – and taking gentle exercise.

breastfeeding nutrition

the nutrients you need

...additional energy intake over and above pre-pregnancy intakes is needed during lactation.

As a guide to a healthy diet during the breastfeeding period, take a look at the nutrients that the British Department of Health recommends. For more information about the nutrients mentioned below, *see* pages 40–61.

Breastfeeding is an energy-demanding activity. Even taking into account the fact that body fat stored during pregnancy is used to supply some of that energy, additional energy intake over and above pre-pregnancy intakes is needed during lactation.

As soon as weaning begins, a mother's energy needs start to return to her pre-pregnancy levels. For the purpose of setting estimated average requirements (EARs), breastfeeding mothers are classified in two groups. Group 1 mothers are those whose breast milk supplies all or most of the infant's food for the first three months only. Group 2 mothers are those who supply all or nearly all the infant's energy and nutrient needs for six months or more (*see* table below).

As soon as weaning begins, a mother's energy needs start to return to her pre-pregnancy levels.

stage of breastfeeding	additional EAR	
Up to one month	450 kcal/day	
1–2 months	530 kcal/day	
2–3 months	570 kcal/day	
	Group 1	**Group 2**
4–6 months	480 kcal/day	570 kcal/day
More than 6 months	240 kcal/day	550 kcal/day

protein

The normal reference nutrient intake (RNI) for protein is:

15- to 18-year olds: 45 g per day
19- to 50-year olds: 45 g per day
over 51: 46 g per day

These amounts increase for lactating women:

up to six months: an additional 11 g per day;

six months and over: an additional 8 g per day.

vitamin A (retinol)

The RNI for women is 600 mg per day, with an additional 350 mg per day for lactating women, totalling 950 mg per day.

vitamin B$_2$ (riboflavin)

The RNI for non-pregnant women is 1.1 mg per day, with an increase of 0.5 mg per day for lactating women, totalling 1.6 mg per day.

vitamin B$_{12}$ (cyanocobalamine)

The RNI for non-pregnant and pregnant women is 1.5 mg per day – a very small amount. The average intake for women in the UK is 5.4 mg, so few women are likely to be deficient. The RNI for lactating women is 2.0 mg per day.

vitamin B$_3$ (niacin)

Lactating women need additional niacin to maintain adequate levels in breast milk. Over and above the increase that will occur as a result of increasing their energy intake.

vitamin C

The RNI for non-pregnant women is 40 mg per day. This increases to 70 mg per day during breastfeeding.

vitamin D

Because sufficient vitamin D is obtained from sunlight, no recommended intake has been set for dietary sources of vitamin D for non-pregnant women. However, lower levels of vitamin D have been found in placentas. Therefore, to avoid low levels in babies, it is recommended that pregnant and breastfeeding women should have a minimum of 10 mg of vitamin D every day.

calcium

The recommended calcium intake for women is 700 mg per day, with an increase to 1,250 mg for lactating women and 1,350 mg for teenage lactating mothers.

magnesium

The RNI for magnesium is 270 mg per day for women. Lactating women need an extra 50 mg per day, totalling 320 mg per day. Teenage lactating mothers need an extra 30 mg per day.

zinc

The dietary requirement for zinc for non-pregnant women is 7 mg per day. This amount increases for lactating women:

0-4 months: plus 6 mg per day
over 4 months: plus 2.5 mg per day.

copper

The RNI for non-pregnant women is 1.2 mg per day, with an addition of 0.3 mg per day for lactating women, totalling 1.5 mg per day.

selenium

The RNI for non-pregnant women is 60 mg per day, with an extra 15 mg per day for lactating women, totalling 75 mg per day.

folate

The RNI for non-pregnant women is 200 ug per day, with an extra 60 ug per day for lactacting women.

"Eat when you're hungry" and "drink when you're thirsty" are the most important points to remember about nutrition and breastfeeding.

The international charity La Leche League International was formed over 40 years ago in the USA, and now has over 3,000 groups meeting in 62 countries, including the UK. It is involved with local health trust breastfeeding working groups, giving advice to the British Food Standards Agency and providing information and support to any mother wishing to breastfeed.

It is a fabulous source of information and has put together many leaflets. "Common breastfeeding myths" is just one that is particularly impressive. Here are a few myths, taken from the leaflet, that La Leche League International can help to dispel. For further details about this charity and other breastfeeding support groups and counsellors, see "Useful Addresses", page 143.

myth: If a baby isn't gaining weight, it may be due to the low quality of the mother's milk.
fact: Studies have shown that even malnourished women are able to produce milk of sufficient quality and quantity to support a growing infant. Most cases of low weight gain are related to insufficient milk intake or an underlying health problem in the baby (*Ref. 5.5*).

myth: Poor milk supply is usually caused by stress, fatigue, and/or inadequate fluids and food intake.
fact: The most common causes of milk supply problems are infrequent feedings and/or poor latch-on and positioning; both are usually due to inadequate information provided to the breastfeeding mother. Suckling problems on the infant's part can also adversely affect milk supply. Stress, fatigue, and malnutrition are rarely causes of milk-supply failure because the body has highly developed survival mechanisms to protect the baby during times of scarce food supply (*Ref. 5.6*).

myth: Some babies are allergic to their mother's milk.

fact: Human milk is the most natural and physiologic substance that a baby can ingest. If a baby shows sensitivities related to feedings, it is usually a foreign protein that has been "piggy-backed" into the mother's milk, and not the milk itself. This is usually handled by removing the offending food from the mother's diet (*Ref. 5.7*).

It is best that substances such as caffeine and chocolate, which contains theobromine, are consumed in moderation.

breastfeeding myths

references

chapter 1

1.1 Old Testament, Judges 13, 3-4 & Barnes, Bradley *Planning for a Healthy Baby* (Vermilion 1994)

1.2 Stewart M. *Healthy Parents, Healthy Baby.* London: Headline, 1995.

1.3 Wynn, A and M *"Prevention of Handicap of Early Pregnancy Origin Today – Building Tomorrow International Conference on Physical Disabilities"*, Montreal 4-6 June 1986; Antonov, A N J *Paediatrics* 30: 250-259 1974 *Children born during the siege of Leningrad in 1942*; Smith, G A J *Paediatrics* 30: 250-259 1974 *"Effects of Maternal Undernutrition Upon the New-born Infant in Holland"*

1.4 Glenville, Marilyn PhD *Natural Solutions to Infertility: How to Increase Your Chances of Conceiving and Preventing Miscarriage* (Judy Piatkus Ltd 2000)

1.5 Refior, Tiffany About.com. www.vegetarian.about.com/food/vegetaria n/library/weekly/aa011700a.htm

1.6 Brown, Judith E *Nutrition and Pregnancy: A Complete Guide from Preconception to Postdelivery* (NTC/Contemporary Publishing Company November 1998)

1.7 Srivastava, K C et al *Danish Medical Bulletin* vol 28 1981, pp 201-3 *"Prostaglandin E and 19-hydroxy-prostaglandin E Content in the Semen of Men with Normal Sperm Characteristics, Men with Abnormal Sperm Characteristics, Vasectomized, and Polyzoospermic Men"*

1.8 Davies, S Zinc *1984-1985 Yearbook of Nutritional Medicine* pp. 113-52 *"Nutrition and Health"* Bland, E (ed) (Keats Publishing, New Canaan, Connecticut 1985)

1.9 *Preparation for Pregnancy*, Bradley, Bennett, publ. Argyll Publishing 1997

1.10 Schwabe, J W R and Rhodes, D *Trends in Biochemical Science*, vol 16 1991, pp 291-6 *"Beyond Zinc Fingers: Steroid Hormone Receptors Have a Novel Structure Motif for DNA Recognition"*

1.11 Hurley, L S *Physiological Reviews* vol 61 1991 pp 249-95 *"Tratogenic Aspects of Manganese, Zinc, and Copper Nutrition"*

1.12 Krznjavi H et al, *Selenium and fertility in men, Trace Elements in Medicine*, vol 9(2) 1992 pp 107-8.

1.13 Kumamoto Y et al, *Clinical efficacy of mecobalamin in treatment of oligospermia*. Results of a double-blind comparative clinical study, Alta Urological Japonica, vol 34 (1988) pp 1109-32.

1.14 Jane Clarke's *Bodyfoods for life*, publ. Seven Dials 1999 p.215

1.15 Fraga C G et al, *Ascorbic acid protects against endogenous oxidative DNA damage in human sperm*, Proceedings of the National Academy of Science, vol 88 (1991) pp 11003-6.

1.16 Dawson E B et al, *Effect of ascorbic acid on male fertility*, Annals of New York Academy of Science, vol 498 1987 pp 812-28.

1.17 Rushton D H et al, letter to Ferritin and fertility, Lancet, vol 337 (1991) p 1554.

1.18 Jane Clarke *Bodyfoods for Life*, publ. Seven Dials 1999

1.19 Bradley, Bennett, *Preparation for Pregnancy*, Argyll 1997

1.20 Foresight Association *see* Useful Addresses

1.21 Lodge Rees E, "Trace Elements in Health" Editor, J. Rose, London, Butterworths 1983

1.22 Bryce-Smith D and Waldron H A, *Lead pollution, disease and behaviour*, Community Health, vol 6 1974 pp 168-75.

1.23 Needleman, Herbert L et al. JAMA 1984 251 (22) and Lacranjan I, *Reproductive ability of workmen occupationally exposed to lead*, Arch Environ Health 1975 20

1.24 Rowland A S et al, *The effect of occupational exposure to mercury vapour on the fertility of female dental assistants*, Occupational and Environmental Medicine, vol 51(1) 1994, pp 28-34.

1.25 Bennett H S et al, *Breast and prostate in men who die of cirrhosis of the liver*, American Journal of Clinical Pathology, vol 20 1950, pp 814-28.

1.26 Ellen Levine *Good Advice From Good Housekeeping*, www.homearts.com

1.27 Glenville, Marilyn *as before* (1.4)

1.28 Jick H et al, *Relation between smoking and age of natural menopause*, Lancet vol 1 1977, pp 1354-5.

1.29 Stewart M *as before* (1.2)

1.30 Himmelberger D U et al, *Cigarette smoking during pregnancy and the occurrence of spontaneous abortion and congenital abnormality*, American Journal of Epidemiology, vol 108 1998 pp 470-79.

1.31 Barnes, Bradley *as before* (1.1)

chapter 2

2.1 Rice, R., *'Fish and healthy pregnancy: more than just a red herring'*, *Professional Care of Mother and Baby*, vol 6(6) (1996), pp. 171-3.

2.2 Reese, M.S. et al, *'Maternal and Parental Long-Chain Fatty Acids: Possible roles in preterm birth'*, American Journal of Obstetrics and Gynecology, vol 176(4) (1997), pp. 907-14.

2.3 Wharton, 1992

2.4 Jameson, 1976

2.5 Doyle et al., 1990

2.6 Doyle et al., 1990

2.7 The US Institute of Medicine, report on Nutrition during Pregnancy 1990

2.8 Doyle, Wendy. *Healthy Eating for Pregnancy*. Hodder & Stoughton 1995 pp.35.

2.9 Department of Health (1992) *Folic Acid and the Prevention of Neural Tube Defects*.

2.10 Milunsky, A. et al., *"Multiviamin/ folic acid supplementation in early pregnancy reduces the prevalence of neural tube defects"* JAMA 262:20, P2847-2852 Nov. 24, 1989.

2.11 Department of Health 1992 *Folic Acid and the Prevention of Neural Tube Defects*.

2.12 Rothman et al, New England Journal of Medicine, vol 333(21) 1995, pp. 157-9.

chapter 3

3.1 Eisenberg, Murkoff,Hathaway, *What to Expect When You're Expecting*, publ. Simon & Schuster

3.2 Holford, Patrick *The Better Pregnancy Diet* Piatkus 1987

3.3 Holford, Patrick (*as before* 3.2)

3.4 Wynn A & Wynn M, *The need for nutritional assessment in the treatment of the infertile patient*, J. Nutr. Med. 1: pp 315-324, 1990

3.5 BabyCenter, Inc www.babycenter.com

3.6 iVillage Inc, iVillage/ParentsPlace.com www.parentsplace.com

3.7 BabyCenter, Inc, www.babycentre.co.uk/general/4444html

3.8 Mother&Baby.co.uk, Emap Digital Limited,www.motherandbaby.co.uk

3.9 Holford, Patrick (*as before* 3.2)

3.10 BabyCenter, Inc www.babycenter.com

3.11 Furuhashi, Nobuaki et al, *Effects of Caffeine Ingestion During Pregnancy*, Gynecologic and Obstetric Investigation, 1985, 19, 187-191

3.12 Infante-Rivard C, Fernandez A, Gauthier R, Rivard G E, *Fetal loss*

associated with caffeine intake before and during pregnancy. Jnl.Am.Med.Ass. 270 (24): 2940-3, 1993

3.13 Stewart M, *as before* (1.2)

3.14 Mosher W D and Pratt W F, *Reproductive impairment in married couples*. United States Vital and Health Statistics: National Survey of Family Growth, Series 23, No 11, 1987

3.15 Koller S, *Pisikofaktoren der Schwangerschaft*, Heidelberg:Springer-Verlag, 1983

chapter 5

5.1 American Academy of Pediatrics, *Policy Statement on Breastfeeding and the Use of Human Milk* (*see* Useful addresses)

5.2 Stigler U, *Preventive dietary management prenatal, neonatal and in infancy*. Clin Ecol, 1985;3:1:50-54

5.3 H and M Diamond, *Fit for Life II: Living Health*, Bantam, London 1987

5.4 Ruth Lawrence MD

5.5 Nancy Mohrbacher 1997; 116-32; Wilde 1995, 401-6.

5.6 Dusdieker 1990, 737-40; Hill 1992, 605-13; Woolridge 1995; World Health Organisation, 1995.

5.7 Hudson 1995, 886-92; Mohrbacher 1997, 97-99; Salmon 1994, 32-33

useful addresses

Foresight Association for the Promotion of Preconceptual Care
28 The Paddock, Godalming, Surrey, GU7 1XD
Tel 01483 427839
Fax 01483 427668

The Active Birth Centre
25 Bickerton Road, London, N19 5JT
Tel 020 7482 5554
Fax 020 7267 9683

National Childbirth Trust (NCT)
Alexandra House, Oldham Terrace, Acton, London, W3 6NH
Tel 020 8992 8639
Fax 020 8992 5929

La Leche League (GB)
BM 1424, London, WC1 3XX
Tel 020 7242 1278

Action on Smoking and Health (ASH)
102 Clifton Street, London, EC2A 4HW
Tel 020 7739 5902
Fax 020 7613 0531

Tommy's Campaign
1 Kennington Road, London,SE1 7RR
Tel 020 7620 0188
Fax 020 7928 6628

The American Academy of Pedriatrics
141 Northwest Point Blvd, Elk Grove Village, IL 60007-1098 USA
Tel 00 1 847 434 4000
Fax 00 1 847 434 8000

acknowledgements

For Jasmine Jade

So many people have provided information for this book that it would be impossible to thank them all. However, I must mention Becca and Emma at Mitchell Beazley for helping to turn my ideas into reality, and Phil, Miranda, and Bill for making the book look so gorgeous. A big thank you goes to James for his extensive research and for coping with the many late nights and weekends, Tanya for her nutrition advice, and Lizzie and Fiona for their assistance. And as always thank you to David, Pop, and Vicki for their continued support.

For everyone planning a family – hope this helps!

index

alcohol 9, 19, 29, 49, 50, 53, 77, 85, 86
allergies 74-5
anaemia 19, 20, 48, 51, 55, 56, 82
antioxidants 18, 21, 23, 27, 53, 58, 59

birth defects 10, 18, 29, 30, 31, 50, 56, 57, 59, 85, 86, 87
see also spina bifida
birth weight 16, 31, 44, 50, 52, 53, 78, 85, 87
blood 19, 20, 48, 51, 53, 55, 56
blood sugar levels 15, 42-3, 77
breads, recipes using 98, 102-3, 123, 126-7, 130, 131
breakfasts
  cereals 96-7
  cooked 98-9
  fruit based 91-7, 98
  smoothies 91-3
breastfeeding 134-40
  nutrients required for 49, 138-9
  peanut allergy and 74

caffeine 22, 28, 49, 77, 85
cake and muffin recipes 98, 131
calcium 48-9, 50, 52, 84
  breastfeeding requirements 49, 139
  sources of 48, 49, 92, 93, 95, 96, 100, 101, 107, 114, 117, 122, 123, 125, 128, 130
carbohydrates 15, 42-3, 53, 54
complex carbohydrates 15, 42, 43, 102, 111, 120
  sources of 42, 43, 104, 110, 118, 124
cereals 96-7, 129
cheese 67
  recipes 100, 101, 102, 107, 108, 123, 127
conception, preparation for 8-31
constipation 14, 82
contraceptive coil 27
contraceptive pill 16, 19, 25, 27, 50
copper 16, 27, 139
cramps 84
cravings 81
curry, recipes 117, 122

desserts 124-5
digestion 36, 46, 53, 97
dressings, sauces and relish 95, 102, 103, 104, 105, 106, 107, 114, 121
drinks 76, 77, 80, 85, 85-6, 93, 129
  with caffeine and tannin (coffee, tea & cola) 22, 28, 53, 77, 85
  herbal teas 85
  soya drink 55, 60, 91, 92, 96, 97
drugs 31
  fertility 27
  pharmaceutical 19, 31, 85
  safety aspects 85-7

eggs 69, 99
energy, nutrition 15, 20, 41, 43, 44, 46, 53, 55, 58
essential fatty acids (EFAs) 12-13, 44-5
exercise 31

fats 12-13, 35, 44-5, 54, 75, 98, 104
  sources of essential fatty acids 45, 103, 105, 118, 126, 128
fertility
  nutrition and 10-25
  what to avoid 26-31
  what to eat 12-25
fibre 14, 92, 95, 97, 100, 102, 103, 107, 109, 112, 126, 130, 131
fish
  fresh and frozen 35, 47, 51, 55, 71
  minerals from 17, 18, 50
  oily 13, 17, 20, 35, 45, 49, 50, 54, 55, 59, 60, 61, 103
  recipes 98, 102, 103, 104, 106, 116-19, 126
  toxins in 27, 71
  see also seafood
folate 101
folic acid
  nutritional value of 19, 51, 53, 55, 56-7, 82, 86
  sources of 19, 91, 95, 96, 98, 100, 105, 106, 107, 108, 117, 122
  see also vitamins
food additives 28, 38, 77
food poisoning 65-6, 69
food sensitivities 36, 74-5
foods
  convenience foods 73
  dealing with discomfort 76-84
  GM free 38
  non-organic 39
  organic 11, 24, 37, 38-9
  processed 43
  raw 36, 37
  safety aspects 64-75
fruit
  breads 130, 131
  breakfasts 91-7, 98
  dried 17, 50, 51, 52, 54, 95, 97, 129
  fibre from 14
  fresh 15, 18, 19, 20, 21, 23, 35, 36, 37, 43, 52, 57, 58, 59, 61, 77
  in soup 109

ginger 76, 115, 122, 129

haemorrhoids 82
hormonal changes 80, 81, 82, 87
hygiene, food and 64-5

indigestion 80
insomnia 83
iron 22, 51, 56, 58, 82
  sources of 51, 75, 95, 96, 99, 101, 106, 113, 122, 125, 127

listeria 65, 67, 70, 72, 73
lunches 100-11
  salads 104-7
  sandwiches 102-3
  soups 108-9
  wraps 100-1

magnesium 48, 50, 52, 84, 106, 123, 124, 125, 139
manganese 18, 82
meat
  liver 59, 60, 70
  recipes 104, 112-15
  safety aspects of 70
medication see drugs, pharmaceutical
milk and cream 68, 92, 96, 97, 136
minerals 16-18, 22, 48-52, 92, 112, 115
  the pill and 25, 50
miscarriage 9, 18, 31, 85, 87
morning sickness 76-7, 115, 122, 129
muffin and cake recipes 98, 131

nausea 76-7
nutrition
  breastfeeding and 138-9
  fertility and 10-25
  pregnancy and 34-61
nuts 74-5, 96, 97, 107, 129
peanuts 20, 50, 53, 74-5

oils 13, 23, 35, 44, 45, 61

pain-killers, caffeine in 28, 85
pets, hygiene and food safety 65
phosphorus 48, 49, 50, 84, 102, 127
phytochemicals 37
piles 82
pizzas 110
potassium 124, 125, 127, 131
poultry, recipes 112, 114-15
preconception care 8-31
pregnancy
  diet during 34-61
  food safety during 64-75
  preparation for 8-31
protein 15, 46-7, 53, 54, 55, 75
  breastfeeding requirements 139
  sources of 46, 47, 91, 92, 96, 97, 99, 100, 107, 108, 109, 112, 113, 114, 115, 117, 118, 119, 123, 126
  vegetarian 47, 54, 92, 96, 97, 100, 108, 109, 112, 122, 123, 126
puddings 124-5

reference nutrient intake (RNI) 40-1

salads 19, 35, 72, 104-7
salmonella 66, 69
seafood see fish
selenium 18, 139
shellfish see fish

smoking 9, 27, 30, 58, 77, 87
  and alcohol 29, 85, 86
snacks 35, 126-9
soups, recipes 108-9
soya drink 55, 60, 91, 92, 96, 97
soya protein 47, 54
spina bifida 19, 56, 57
  see also birth defects
sugars 15, 35, 42-3, 77
suppers 112-23
  fish 116-19
  meat & poultry 112-15
  vegetarian 120-3
supplements
  minerals 77
  vitamins 19, 55, 57, 61, 77, 87

teeth and bones 48, 52, 60
tortillas 100, 101, 110
toxic metals 18, 26-7, 71
toxins
  environmental 24, 27, 38, 85
  in fish 27, 71
  nausea and 77
  reproductive system and 14
toxoplasmosis 66, 68, 70, 72

vegan diets 11, 15, 20, 49, 55
  recipes 91, 93, 94-5, 97, 103, 105, 108, 109, 111, 122
vegetables, roasted 113, 120
vegetarian diets 11, 15, 47
  recipes 91-7, 108-11, 120-3
vitamins 19-23, 37, 44, 49, 52-5, 92
  A (beta-carotene/retinol) 21, 50, 52, 53, 59, 60, 70, 86, 91, 93, 99, 104, 105, 108, 111, 112, 113, 115, 122, 127, 139
  B complex vitamins 52, 53-5, 75, 96, 112, 128
  B1 (thiamine) 53, 86
  B2 (riboflavin) 53, 54, 139
  B3 (niacin/nicotinic acid) 53, 54, 139
  B5 (pantothenic acid) 53
  B6 (pyridoxine) 20, 50, 53, 55, 77, 82
  B12 (cobalamin/cyanocobalamine) 20, 53, 55, 82, 139
  C 21, 22, 27, 51, 52, 53, 58, 60, 91, 93, 95, 102, 103, 104, 106, 107, 110, 111, 113, 115, 118, 120, 123, 126, 139
  D 49, 52, 59, 60, 61, 139
  E 23, 50, 52, 53, 60, 61, 107, 110, 127
  K 52
  see also folic acid

weight 25, 78-9

zinc 16-17, 27, 29, 50, 77, 86
  breastfeeding requirements 139
  sources of 17, 50, 96, 123, 128